The Little Book of Crystals

Crystals to attract love, wellbeing, and spiritual harmony into your life

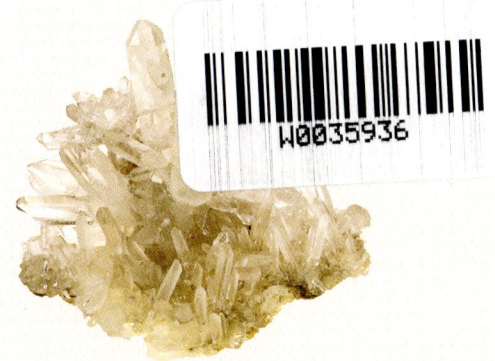

Judy Hall

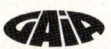

An Hachette UK Company
www.hachette.co.uk

First published in Great Britain in
2016 by Gaia, a division of Octopus
Publishing Group Ltd,
Carmelite House,
50 Victoria Embankment,
London EC4Y 0DZ
www.octopusbooks.co.uk

Distributed in the US by Hachette
Book Group, 1290 Avenue of the
Americas, 4th and 5th Floors,
New York, NY 10104

Distributed in Canada by Canadian
Manda Group, 664 Annette St.,
Toronto, Ontario, Canada M6S 2C8

ISBN 978-1-85675-361-6

A CIP catalogue record for this book
is available from the British Library.

Printed and bound in China

10 9 8 7

Commissioning Editor
Leanne Bryan
Editor Pollyanna Poulter
Art Director Juliette Norsworthy
Designer Isabel de Cordova
Illustrations Abigail Read
Production Controller
Allison Gonsalves

Disclaimer
No medical claims are made for the stones in
this book and the information given is not
intended to act as a substitute for medical
treatment. The healing properties are given
for guidance only and are, for the most
part, based on anecdotal evidence and/
or traditional therapeutic use. If in any
doubt, a crystal healing practitioner should
be consulted. In the context of this book,
illness is a disease, the final manifestation
of spiritual, environmental, psychological,
karmic, emotional or mental imbalance or
distress. Healing means bringing mind, body
and spirit back into balance and facilitating
evolution for the soul; it does not imply
a cure. In accordance with crystal healing
consensus, all stones are referred to as
crystals regardless of whether or not they
have a crystalline structure.

The Little
Book of
Crystals

Contents

INTRODUCTION

Are you drawn to bright, sparkling
gemstones? Ones that have been faceted —
cut to display flat, polished surfaces —
to show them off in the best light? Most
people are. But do you ever look at a
rough lump of rock labelled "crystal"
and wonder what all the fuss is about?

Crystals can look very dull — until you feel their energy.
Crystals don't have to be big and blingy to be powerful.
A small, raw chunk of crystal can work as well as a large,
polished one. Most crystals in this book will be in any
crystal shop, although one or two (the more unusual,
new high-vibration stones — those that work at a higher
frequency) may have to be obtained from an online store.
They are worth seeking out, and that is why they have
been included. As you will discover, crystals have definite
personalities of their own, and these key players insisted
that they should meet you.

*Barnacle Bridge Quartz has
many external shapes, but
one crystal underneath.*

What is a crystal?

A crystal is a solid substance with a geometrically regular internal lattice, with faces and axes that may or may not be reflected in its external shape. It is formed from one of seven possible geometric forms: triangles, squares, rectangles, hexagons, rhomboids, parallelograms, or trapeziums (trapezoids). These forms lock together into a variety of three-dimensional crystal shapes. It is this inner structure that defines the type of crystal.

Each type of crystal is made from its own particular mineral and chemical recipe, which affects its colour. In crystal healing, amorphous crystals that cooled too fast to crystallize, or that were created from events such as a meteorite hitting the Earth, may not have a repeating internal atomic crystal structure, but are nevertheless referred to as crystals.

Crystal benefits

People who regularly use crystals report benefits such as:

◊ Peace and tranquillity
◊ An increased sense of wellbeing and enhanced immunity
◊ Mental clarity and focus
◊ The feeling of being in a safe, sacred space
◊ High energy and a zest for life
◊ Less depression and anxiety, and more joy
◊ Reduced pain and muscle tension
◊ Guidance and insight

Crystal history

Crystals were an essential part of
the ancient world and were integral to
magic, religion, and mystery. From the
beautifully crafted flint and jade ritual
axes of the early Stone Age to the
intricate jewellery worn by the pharaohs,
crystals appeared everywhere.

Crystals are mentioned 1,704 times in the Bible, so don't
ever let anyone tell you they are a nutty "New Age"
invention – or "ungodly". There were certainly crystals on
the famous Breastplate of the High Priest created by Moses
for his brother Aaron.

In India, China, Mesopotamia, Greece, and Egypt
crystals were used for ritual and medicinal purposes and
were part of the earliest scientific treatises. In prehistoric
times some crystals were traded thousands of miles: Lapis
Lazuli was transported from high in the Afghan mountains
to Egypt and beyond and 9,000 years ago, Baltic Amber
was carried in the opposite direction.

Crystals have been revered, lusted after, fought over, and
bought for extortionate sums for millennia. And gemstones
continue to form a part of royal regalia and symbols of
power worldwide.

Crystal power

What were the mysterious, magical powers that crystals embodied? In ancient times crystals were regarded as divine and were used for both healing and protection – a practice that continues today in addition to being used to run computers and power the lasers that are used in surgery.

Energy patterns

Crystals have a stable and unchanging energy pattern, and each crystal has a unique frequency and energy field, or resonance. They act like tuning forks, bringing the energies around them into harmony. Our bodies have very unstable energy fields and any disruption creates "dis-ease", but if you put the stable energy field of a crystal alongside a disorganized human field, the energies entrain – come together – and the disharmonious field is brought back to its pristine form. Harmony and wellbeing are the result.

Jade was used in China as a symbol of good fortune for thousands of years.

Energy generators

Some crystals actually create energy. Pyroelectric crystals generate electricity when heated or cooled. When early humans struck two flints together to create a spark to light a fire, they created electricity. Greek philosopher Theophrastus (c.372–287BCE) noted that Tourmaline attracted and repelled straw due to an electrostatic charge.

You don't need to heat a crystal to create energy. Quartz under pressure generates electricity, known as piezoelectricity. The process was discovered by brothers Pierre (1859–1906) and Paul-Jacques Curie (1856–1941) in the 1880s. Piezoelectric crystals transform mechanical action into electricity, or electricity into mechanical action – and the energy is stable. So Quartz converts the electrical charge in a battery into a steady beat that regulates a watch. It is also used in cigarette and gas lighters, the buzzers found in microwave ovens and phones, minute microphones and earphones, and inkjet printers.

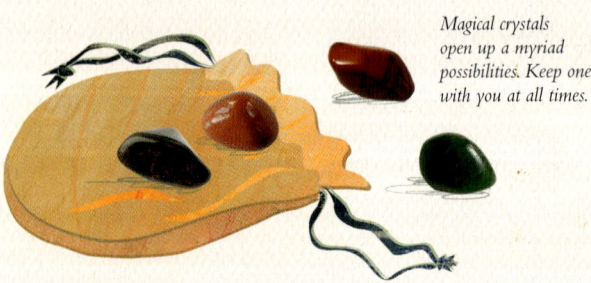

Magical crystals open up a myriad possibilities. Keep one with you at all times.

Crystal attributes

The internal structure, composition, and properties of a crystal determine its crystal family. But colour and shape affect how the energy of a crystal manifests.

Crystal colour

The colour of a crystal is in the eye of the beholder. Light is split and refracted and perceived as energy by the eye and as colour by the brain.

Crystal colours and what they signify

- Silver-grey: Transmutation; traditionally imparts invisibility
- Black: Protection and grounding; excellent detoxifier
- Brown: Cleansing and purification; centredness
- Pink: Lovingness; alleviates anxiety, dispels trauma
- Peach: Gentle energizing
- Red: Energizing and activating
- Orange: Vibrant vitality, creativity, and assertiveness
- Yellow: Clarity, wealth, and abundance
- Green: Calmness, emotional healing, compassion
- Green-blue/turquoise: Intuition, peace, and relaxation
- Blue: Self-expression, communication
- Lavender/lilac/purple: Spiritual realities, intuition
- White: Purity; the highest realms of being
- Clear: Energizing; purification, higher consciousness
- Combination/bicoloured: Synergy, exciting possibilities

Crystal shape

The external shape of a crystal may bear little resemblance to its internal lattice. Crystals may be sharp points, clusters, or flat plates that can be cut and artificially shaped. Its shape affects the way energy – and light – moves through it.

External crystal shapes and what they signify

◇ Ball: Emits energy equally all round

◇ Cluster: Radiates energy in all directions equally

◇ Point: Draws off or pulls in energy, when pointed out or in towards the body

◇ Double-terminated (pointed at both ends): Emits energy in two directions

◇ Egg: Focuses and discharges energy

◇ Geode (a crystal-lined cavity): Amplifies, conserves, and slowly releases energy

◇ Square: Consolidates energy

These properties are used in crystal healing and to create a better environment. With the assistance of your crystal friends, you can transform negative energy into beneficial energy, improve your wellbeing and bring positivity into your life. But first there are a few essential steps to take.

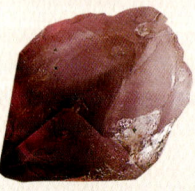

These Amethysts have the same internal structure.

Quick Reference

Before you can enjoy your crystals
fully, there are a few secrets
that you need to know, so we'll
look at how to keep your crystals
energetically clean and working
well for you — and at how you might
programme and use them, once they
are cleansed. You can use your
crystals simply for decoration,
of course, but that is a bit
wasteful of their extraordinary
powers for healing, space-clearing,
and energy-management.

Choosing your crystal

You can choose a crystal described in this book, or you can choose one using your intuition, which is much more fun. Simply by letting your eyes roam over a shelf of crystals, you will find one that calls particularly to you. It will catch your attention and hold it – that is the crystal for you. It may not be the prettiest, or the biggest, but it will be the most potent for you. Treasure it well.

Let your fingers do the choosing

Run your fingers through a tub of tumbled (smoothed and polished) crystals and something amazing happens. One crystal will generally find its way into your hand, and you won't be able to let go of it. This is the stone for you.

If the stones are bigger, then finger-dowsing uses a little-known ability of the human body to attune you to the energies of the crystals and recognize exactly the right frequency for you. How? By using your kinetic senses – the ability to feel energy. Your intuition communicates that knowledge to your fingers.

Finger-dowsing helps you to select the right crystal.

Finger-dowsing crystals

1 Loop your thumb and finger together, as shown.

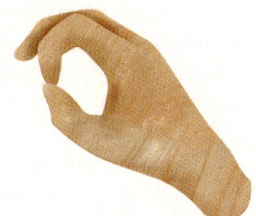

2 Slip your other thumb and finger through the loop and close them together. Hold your hands over a crystal – or a photograph of one – and ask, "Is this the crystal for me?"

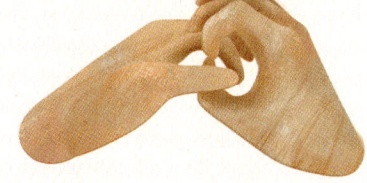

3 If the loop holds, then the answer is "yes". If it pulls apart, the answer is "no".

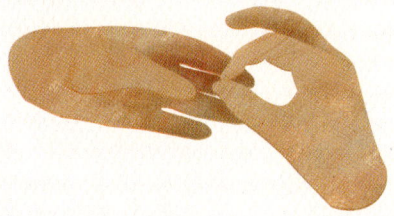

Cleansing your crystal

Crystals pick up the vibration of everyone who has handled them. They also soak up negative energies. If you have just bought a crystal, it will need cleansing. Once you have worn or used it for a while, it will need cleansing again. If you feel dragged down or irritable when wearing a crystal, cleanse it before deciding whether or not it's right for you.

Purifying your crystals

◊ Most crystals can be cleansed and recharged by holding them under running water for a few minutes. Natural water from a stream or the sea is best, but you can use tap water. Put small crystals in a porous bag, to prevent them from being washed away.

◊ Crystals can also be cleansed by being placed in a bowl of salt or brown rice overnight, then brushing off the salt or rice afterwards (salt is best avoided if the crystal is fragile, layered, or friable). They can also be placed on a large Quartz cluster or a Carnelian, then put in the sun for a few hours. If it is not sunny, visualize a bright white light radiating down onto the crystals. White stones benefit from recharging in moonlight.

Alternative cleansing methods

Smudging: Sage, sweetgrass, or joss sticks quickly remove negative energies from crystals. Light the smudge stick (a bundle of dried herbs) or joss stick and pass it over the crystal, if it is large; or hold the crystal in your hand in the smoke, if it is small.

Visualizing light: Hold the crystal in your hands and visualize a column of bright white light coming down and covering it. If you find visualization difficult, use the light of a candle instead and hold the crystal a safe distance above the flame.

Bought remedies: Purpose-made crystal-clearing remedies are available from essence suppliers. Either drop the remedy directly onto the crystal or put a few drops into spring water in a spray bottle, then gently mist the crystal.

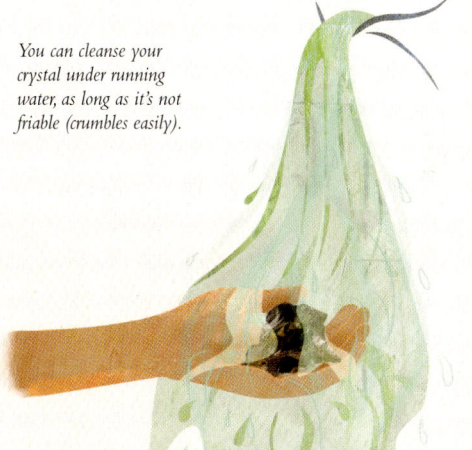

You can cleanse your crystal under running water, as long as it's not friable (crumbles easily).

Programming your crystal

Spending a few moments asking your crystal to work in harmony with you will repay you with a potent and powerful crystal energy.

Activating your crystal

1 Hold the crystal in your hands.
2 Close your eyes and concentrate on the crystal.
3 Visualize it surrounded by bright white light.
4 Ask that your crystal will be blessed by the highest energies in the universe.
5 Ask that it is attuned to your own unique frequency and that it is activated to act for your highest good.
6 Then state your intention for your crystal – for example "This crystal will help me to heal", "This crystal will attract abundance and good fortune to me" – and ask it to work with you in order to achieve it.

Storing your crystal

If you look after your crystals, they will repay you with years of devoted service. A cloth bag can be useful to store tumbled stones, although even these may scratch in time.

Jewellery and more delicate stones – especially those crystals with points – should be kept wrapped in a cloth or displayed on a shelf. A box with divisions, or a bowl, can also be used to store individual stones.

Using your crystal

Crystals can be worn, placed on or around your body, or sited in your environment, to bring healing, safety, peace, relaxation, and motivation. They can also help to reverse the causes of dis-ease, whether at a mental, spiritual, emotional, or physical level.

Feasting your eyes If you have one big, bold, and beautiful crystal, be sure to place it where you will see it frequently. It will radiate all good things to you.

Wearing your crystal
Crystal jewellery is an excellent way to keep crystal vibes with you throughout the day. Wherever possible, wear the crystal against your skin, for maximum benefit.

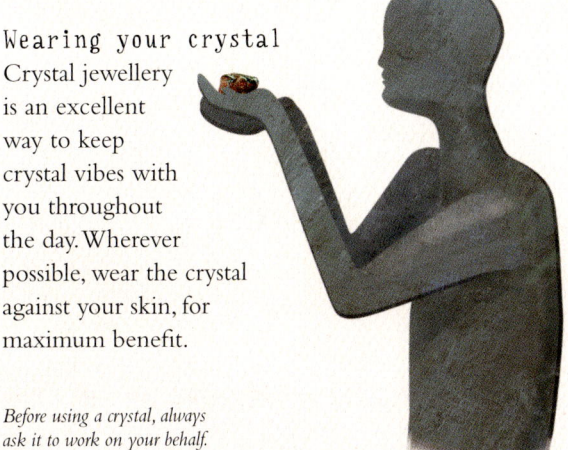

Before using a crystal, always ask it to work on your behalf.

Creating a safe, sacred space Placing your crystals around you in a harmonious pattern creates a safe space and cleanses negativity. Try using Selenite and Black Tourmaline in a Star of David (see below). Place three Black Tourmaline stones at the points of an imaginary triangle, point up, first. Then place three Selenite stones at the points of a second imaginary triangle, point down, over the top. Make the grid either big or small, depending on how much space you have. Even a tiny grid works wonders.

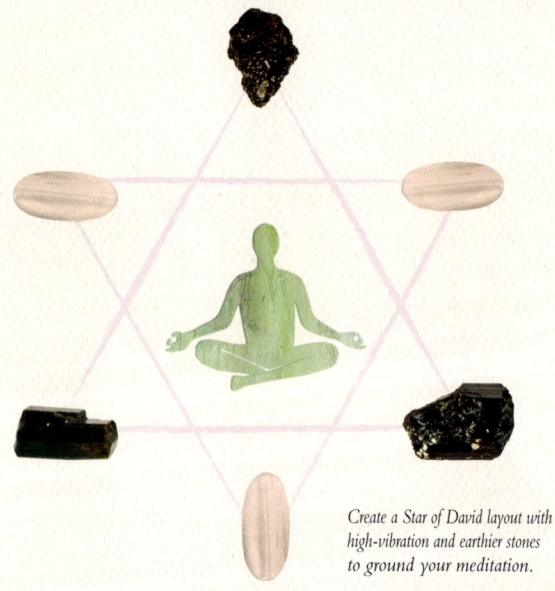

Create a Star of David layout with high-vibration and earthier stones to ground your meditation.

Meditating Sit and gaze into the depths of a crystal, to centre and calm yourself.

Protecting yourself Wear Shungite or Black Tourmaline, or place a selection of crystals on a windowsill or shelf, to protect you and fill your home with good vibes.

Blocking negative or toxic energy Place a large Black Tourmaline or Shungite against a computer or any other source of toxic EMF (electromagnetic force) energy.

Relaxation layout Lie down and place crystals all around your head, pointing inwards, to help you to relax. Amethyst or Auralite 23 is particularly good for this purpose.

Bringing in good vibes Place crystals over and around you in a figure-of-eight, with high-vibration stones such as Selenite, Quartz, or Anandalite™ on the top half, and Red Jasper or Smoky Quartz on the bottom half, to anchor them.

Using crystals for healing Dis-ease is a state of disharmony. All dis-ease is ultimately caused by your body being out of balance, whether at the physical, emotional, or mental level (see overleaf). Fortunately, spending time with your crystals will quickly bring your body back into equilibrium and will relax your mind.

Causes of dis-ease

Damaged immune system: Your immune system is your first line of defence against dis-ease. If it's damaged, dis-ease results. **Solution:** Use Shungite in the form of infused water, or place Bloodstone or Jade over the centre of your chest.

Stress and tension: Running on high adrenaline and putting a continual stress on your body will ultimately manifest as a physical illness. **Solution:** Relax! Place Auralite 23 on the middle of the forehead or meditate with Selenite.

Inadequate rest: Overworking, overthinking, and not taking time out to relax can all result in dis-ease. **Solution:** Pop an Amethyst or Auralite 23 under your pillow.

Emotional exhaustion: If you are continually drained – whether by a person or a situation – then you will have lowered resistance to dis-ease. **Solution:** Place Green Aventurine under your left armpit.

Shock or trauma: Following a shock, your body goes out of balance and dis-ease results. **Solution:** Place Rose Quartz over your heart.

Negative attitudes or toxic emotions: Emotions such as guilt or suppressed anger are insidious precursors to dis-ease, as are low self-esteem and shame. **Solution:** Place a Smoky Quartz on your solar plexus (on your abdomen, beneath the diaphragm) and let it drain off the toxic emotions.

Anxiety or fear: Chronic anxiety and continual fear will weaken the body. **Solution:** Snuggle up with an Anandalite™ crystal.

Crystal essences

Crystal essences are an easy and fun way to use the power of these vibrant stones. By immersing the crystal in spring water, the crystal's vibrations are transferred into an easily assimilated form. These energetic essences work at a subtle level to effect change (usually emotional or psychological), and they are excellent space-clearers and energy-enhancers.

Making an essence

1 Cleanse your crystal (see page 16).
2 Place it in a clean glass bowl and cover with pure spring water. (If the crystal is toxic – none of those discussed in this book – layered, soluble, or fragile, place it in an empty, clean glass bowl, then place the bowl in the water.)
3 Leave in sun- or moonlight for 6–12 hours (white stones benefit from moonlight).

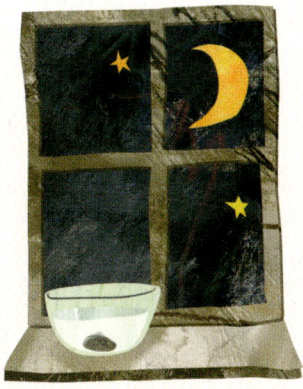

Place your crystal essence in sunshine or moonlight.

4 Remove the crystal and add two-thirds brandy, vodka, or cider vinegar to one-third water as a preservative. (This is the mother tincture and needs dilution before being used.)

Using the crystal essence

1 Add seven drops of mother tincture to a small glass dropper bottle, then top up with one-third brandy and two-thirds water. Sip at regular intervals, rub on the skin, or bathe affected parts of the body.
2 A few drops of gem essence can also be added to a spray bottle of water – add one-quarter vodka or white rum as a preservative, if you are using it over more than a day or two, then spritz it around you, your home, or your workspace. Gem essence can also be dispersed around your aura (the energy field that surrounds the body) by putting a few drops on your hands and then sweeping them from feet to head, about 30cm (12in) away from your body.

Try making

◊ Rose Quartz essence to bathe yourself in love
◊ Red Jasper essence to pep yourself up
◊ Black Tourmaline essence to protect yourself
◊ Jade essence to make you feel so good
◊ Selenite essence to create a sacred space
◊ Smoky Quartz space-clearing essence

Key Crystals

Using just a few key crystals — such
as the ones suggested on the following
pages — will make your life so much
more dynamic. Your crystal friends
will pep you up and add zest to
your life, or will calm you when
necessary. These captivating stones
will also protect you and ensure your
wellbeing. They can take you to new
spiritual heights, or accompany you
through the everyday. They are ideal
for bringing your energies back into
balance and for healing dis-ease.
Just remember to ask your crystal
and state your intention for what you
need from it.

Shungite: Healing

It is believed that Shungite, a rare carbon mineral from outer space, formed when an enormous meteorite crashed into Karelia in northern Russia two billion years ago.

This crystal contains virtually all the minerals in the periodic table, and has phenomenal shielding power that arises from its unique formation. Shungite is composed of fullerenes (hollow carbon molecules), otherwise called "buckyballs". These empower nanotechnology, being excellent geothermal and electromagnetic conductors, and yet they also shield from detrimental electromagnetic frequencies.

Research has shown that Shungite is anti-viral and anti-bacterial, absorbing hazards such as pesticides, free radicals (harmful molecules), and EMF emissions.

Each person has their own unique vibration and bioenergetic field. So there is no "one stone fits all" remedy – although Shungite probably comes closest.
Judy Hall, Crystal Prescriptions, vol.3

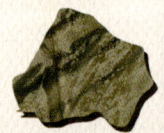

Body: Anecdotal evidence and scientific research suggest that Shungite – a traditional cure-all – strengthens the immune system and assists cellular metabolism. It enhances enzyme production and provides pain relief. A natural detoxifier and anti-inflammatory, it has long been used to encourage wound-healing. Shungite transforms water into a biologically active, life-enhancing substance, while at the same time removing harmful micro-organisms and pollutants.

Note: Shungite water is made differently to a crystal essence (see pages 23-4). Place 100g (3.5oz) of Shungite in a mesh bag. Place the bag in a 1l (35fl oz) jug and fill with spring water. Leave for 48 hours to become biologically active. Drink frequently, topping up the water each time. Cleanse the crystals weekly by running them under the tap and placing in the sun for a few hours.

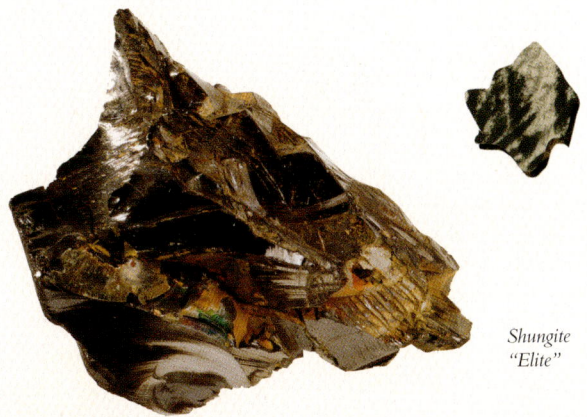

Shungite "Elite"

Physiological correspondences: Immune system, neurotransmitters (nerve-impulse transmitters), cardiovascular, digestive, and filtration systems; kidney and liver, gall-bladder, pancreas.

Mind: Shungite helps you to identify and release old belief patterns, so that fresh patterns can imprint themselves. At the same time it encourages you to recognize the wisdom of the past and apply it to the present, to create a new future.

Place Shungite next to your computer to protect against EMF radiation.

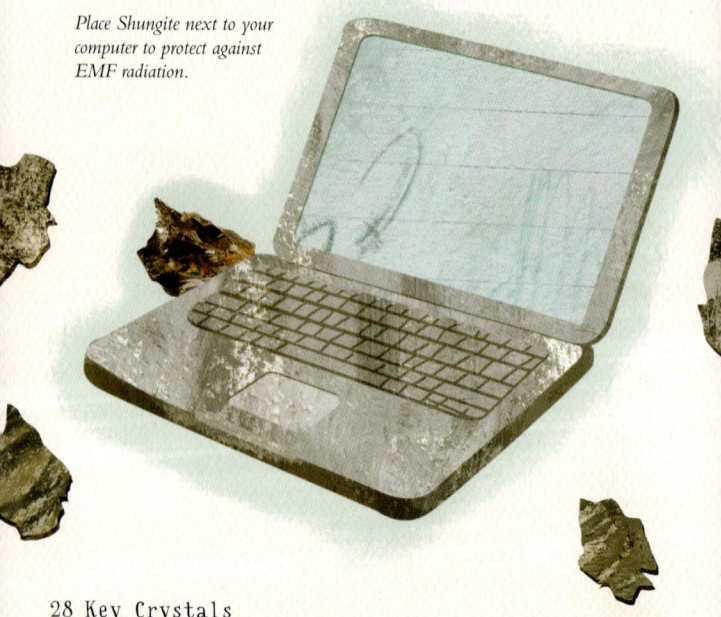

Emotions: Knowing that Shungite has phenomenal shielding power helps you to feel safe within your own skin. Wear it during turbulent times, to reassure yourself and create a tranquil space around you.

Spirit: As this stone came from outer space, it helps you to be aware that you are not alone, and that there is far more to life than you can imagine. It keeps you grounded and protected during meditation and out-of-body journeying.

Curious fact: "Mother Russia is so-called because it was believed that Shungite sowed the seeds of life on Earth," says John Palaguta-Iles (1971–), founder of the Rainbow Chain, which sources Shungite direct from Karelia, Russia.

Did you know? Shungite is created from carbon-based minerals that normally arise from decayed organic matter. However, as there were no forests on Earth at the time, the meteorite that crashed into Karelia must have brought the carbon with it. Shungite water has been used at a healing spa at Lake Onega in Karelia for hundreds of years.

Hot tip: A Shungite pyramid placed by your bed counteracts insomnia and headaches, and eliminates the physiological effects of stress and EMF pollution.

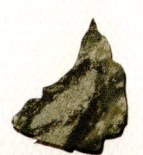
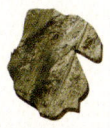

Bloodstone: Body

As its name suggests, Bloodstone has long been regarded as an excellent blood-cleanser and a powerful healer. It was believed to have mystical and magical properties that controlled the weather and conferred the ability to banish evil.

Bloodstone was regarded as a shape-shifting stone because it changed colour in different lights. In the shamanic tradition, it was thought that this crystal taught how to travel invisibly between the worlds and negotiate different realms.

Bloodstone preserves a person's life and keeps him unharmed and bestows a good reputation on those who wear it, and keeps poisons at bay, and all kinds of horrible monsters.
Damigeron, De Virtutibus Lapidum
(The Virtues of Stones)

Body: Found in one of the earliest ever crystal recipes, Bloodstone has long been used to heal blood and blood-rich organs and to encourage good circulation. It stimulates the flow of lymph and the metabolic processes, revitalizing and re-energizing when body and mind are exhausted. In the Middle Ages, Bloodstone was said to stop nosebleeds, and in both the ancient Near East and in the West at this time it was powdered and mixed with honey and egg-white, to draw out snake venom, reduce tumours, and staunch haemorrhages. According to the Lapidary of King Alphonso of Spain, when hung over an abscess, Bloodstone cleared up putrefaction in a day.

Physiological correspondences: Blood and circulation, kidneys, adrenals, liver, gall-bladder, spleen, bladder, intestines, thymus, immune and lymphatic systems; metabolic processes, eyes, detoxification, over-acidification.

Mind: Bloodstone calms the mind. It instils courage, but teaches the value of strategic withdrawal and flexibility. It helps you to recognize that chaos often precedes transformation. This is a perfect stone for mindfulness: focusing your awareness on the present moment, while accepting your thoughts, bodily sensations, and emotions.

Bloodstone is so named because of its red spots.

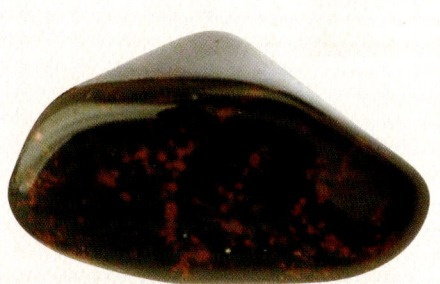

Emotions: Bloodstone helps to calm the heart, reducing emotions such as irritability, aggressiveness, and impatience.

Spirit: Bloodstone facilitates bringing spirituality into everyday life. The stone cleanses and re-energizes the chakras (the energy centres in the body) and the aura.

Curious fact: The Roman geographer Pliny the Elder recorded the belief that Bloodstone had the power to make the moon passing over the disc of the sun visible during an eclipse, but refuted that it conferred invisibility on the wearer.

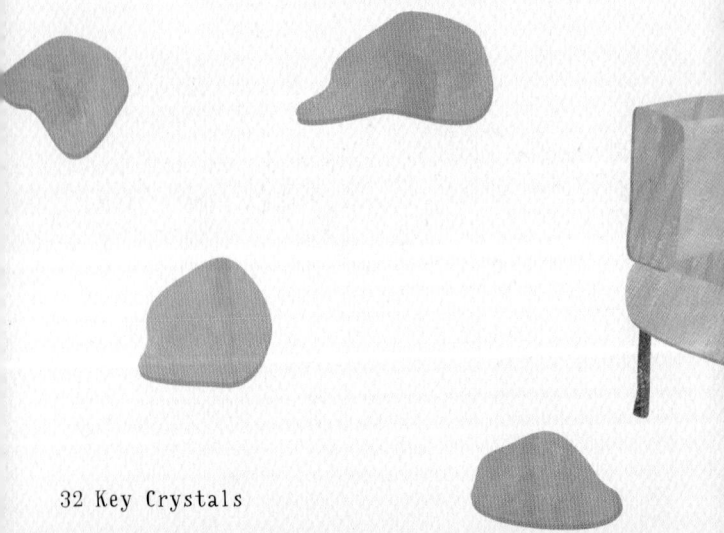

Did you know? In medieval times Christians believed that this stone was created when drops of Christ's blood fell on it at the crucifixion. However, ancient documents record its use as a healing stone three thousand years earlier.

Hot tip: Tape a Bloodstone over your thymus (in the middle of your breastbone) whenever a cold or flu threatens.

A Bloodstone over your thymus stimulates your immune system.

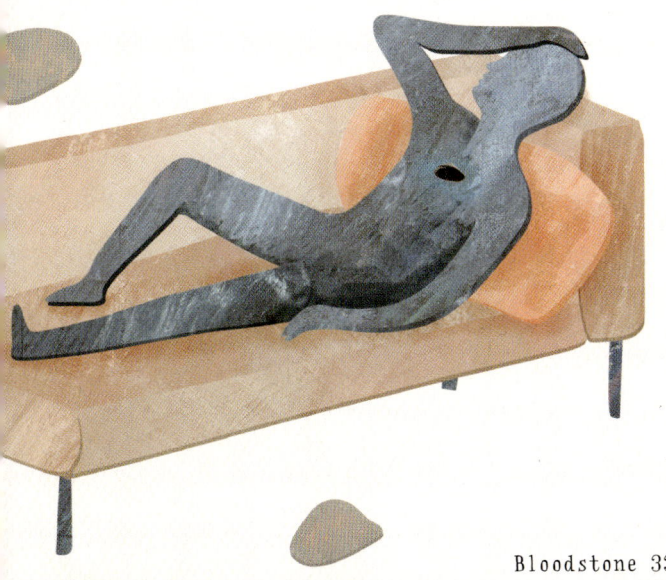

Auralite 23: Mind

Named after the beautiful aurora borealis (Northern Lights phenomenon, which Native Americans call "the Dancing of the Spirits") and after the 23 minerals originally believed to make up this crystal, Auralite 23 – "the Stone of Awakening" – is a unique Amethyst from the Cave of Wonders in Thunder Bay, Canada. Although it can be used on the physical body, its most potent effect is on the mind and spirit. Also called "the paradigm-shifter", it works synergistically with other high-vibration crystals to boost their effect.

Brushing the clouds away from my eyes, I see clarity in the raindrop and beauty in the first ray of morning sun.
Virginia Alison, author of Heaven Scent

Body: Auralite 23's most beneficial physical effect is switching off stress and tension, allowing the body to relax at every level. It clears headaches and migraine, eye strain, muscle spasms, and discomfort. It has also been found to assist vascular health.

Physiological correspondences: The chakras and subtle-energy bodies (namely the biomagnetic, energetic sheath that surrounds the physical body).

Mind: Auralite 23 has a sedative effect, stilling the mind so that conscious connection with higher dimensions occurs. This brings about a mindshift as new awareness opens up. It can literally blow your mind, if you're not prepared for its powerful energetic charge. But, if you are, serenity ensues.

Emotions: Auralite 23 calms the emotions – especially a hot temper – instilling a deep sense of peace. It dissolves the emotional debris that gives rise to psychosomatic "dis-ease".

Auralite 23 is a powerful mind-changer.

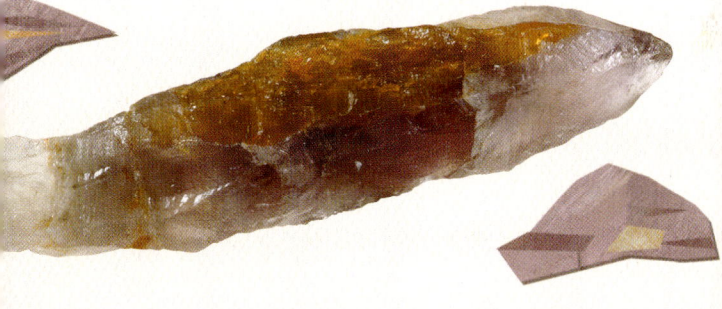

Spirit: This stone gives spiritual growth a powerful kick-start. With its meteoric origins, Auralite 23 forms a bridge to the divine. It deepens meditation and enhances metaphysical abilities. Holding the stone helps you to get in touch with guardian beings and mentors.

Curious fact: Auralite 23 was born 1.2 billion years ago in the Mesoproterozoic age, just as multicellular creatures first emerged on the Earth and began to flourish. It is believed that meteoric strikes brought rare minerals to the Earth's surface to combine and form this multicoloured Amethyst.

Did you know? Testing by the Gemological Institute of America revealed that Auralite 23 is a combination of at least 34 different minerals, including Titanite, Cacoxenite, Lepidocrosite, Ajoite, Haematite, Magnetite, Pyrite, Pyrolusite, Gold, Silver, Platinum, Nickel, Copper, Iron, Limonite, Sphalerite, Covellite, Chalcopyrite, Gialite, Epidote, Bornite, Rutile, Titanite, and Smoky Quartz in Amethyst.

Hot tip: If you have a monkey mind that is continually whirling with thoughts, place Auralite 23 in the middle of your forehead, to switch off the chatter and bring you clarity.

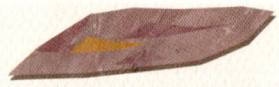

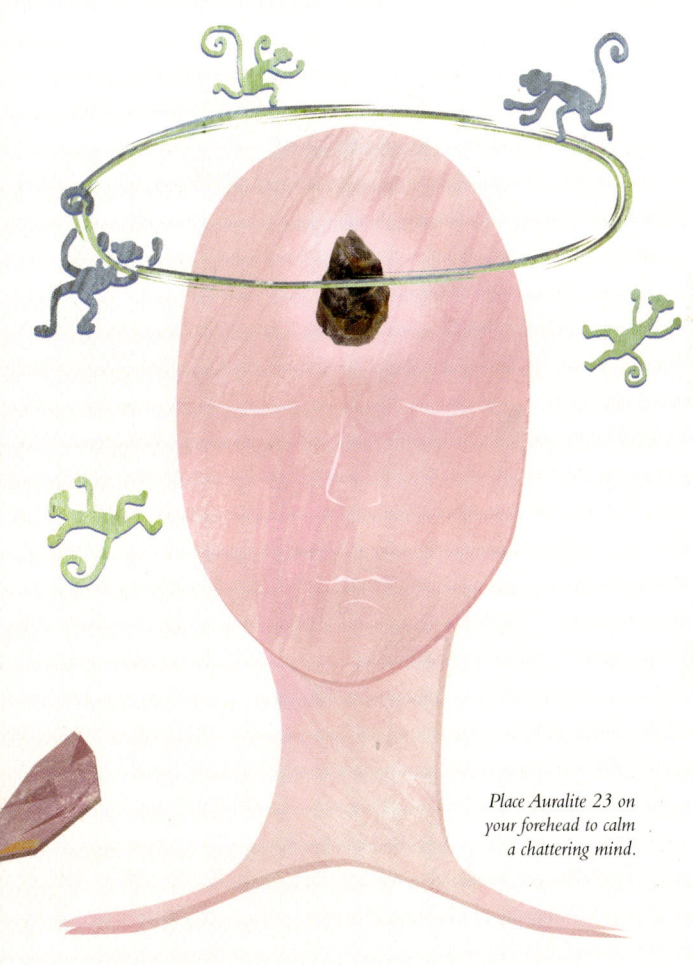

*Place Auralite 23 on
your forehead to calm
a chattering mind.*

Auralite 23 37

Anandalite™ (Aurora Quartz): Spirit

Anandalite (also known as Aurora or Rainbow Quartz) is named after the Sanskrit word ananda, meaning "divine bliss". This stone has some of the highest vibrations yet to be found in the crystal kingdom. It connects you to your soul and beyond.

The crystal facilitates the awakening of kundalini (the life force held at the base of the spine, which can rise up to the head when activated), but if kundalini rises in an undirected, disconnected fashion, it can create imbalances in the physical body. Anandalite smoothes the passage of kundalini up the spine and through the body to release any emotional blockages that stand in the way of spiritual awakening.

A particle of Its bliss supplies the bliss of the whole
universe. Everything becomes enlightened in Its light.
The Vijnanananka

Body: Anandalite opens and aligns all the chakras, dissolving any dis-ease that may have had a psychosomatic effect on the physical body.

Physiological correspondences: Central nervous system, physical and psychic immune system; meridians (energy pathways), chakras, and subtle-energy bodies.

Mind: Anandalite helps you to tune into the infinite possibilities of the higher universal mind – the source of profound wisdom and clarity.

Emotions: This crystal facilitates a gentle, cathartic emotional release and instils profound joy in its place. It is a wonderful stone for lifting depression and anxiety.

*Anandalite is named for
frozen divine light.*

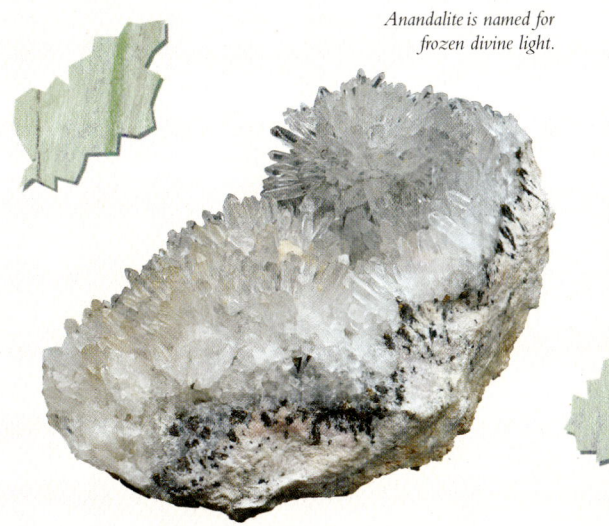

Spirit: Anandalite is a powerful crystal for igniting your spiritual awareness. It immerses you in the quantum field – what the ancients called bliss consciousness, divine light, or enlightenment. It opens the crown and higher crown chakras, to help you tune into your true nature as a child of the universe. This "light-body activation" crystal fills your whole being with light. With it, you will feel connected to the greater divine whole.

Curious fact: The natural iridescent rainbow-flashes on the surface of this Quartz are probably caused by the mineral rhodium, although no one knows for sure.

Did you know? Anandalite purifies the chakras and opens the way for kundalini energy to rise up your spine and into your head – but only when you have prepared the way! Asking for guidance from an experienced crystal and kundalini practitioner is recommended. Kundalini is a wild force that needs guiding with care.

Hot tip: To spring-clean your aura and chakras, sweep Anandalite from your toes up over your head and down your back, then all the way back again.

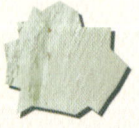
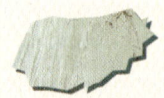
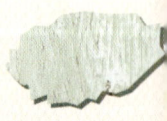

*Sweep Anandalite
all around your body
to cleanse your aura.*

Jade: Health and wellbeing

In ancient times Jade was prized in China, where it was believed to attract good luck and friendship and ensure safety from harm. In the West it was shaped into ceremonial axeheads. A soapy stone found in two forms, Jadeite and Nephrite, it is still used today to attract abundance and ensure wellbeing. It is associated with the heart chakra, and increases love and the capacity to nurture yourself.

> *Jade is precious not because it is rarer, but because the quality of jade... corresponds to such virtues as benevolence, wisdom, righteousness, propriety, loyalty, and trustworthiness... The noble virtues are the manifestation of heavenly principles.*
> *Confucius (551–479*BCE*),*
> *Chinese philosopher*

Body: Jade is a cleansing stone, assisting the body's filtration and elimination organs and supporting the immune system. Crystal healers use it to rebind the cellular and skeletal systems. It has long been believed that Jade detoxifies the kidneys and balances bodily fluids and the ratio of water to salt and acid to alkaline. This crystal is traditionally used to assist fertility and childbirth.

Physiological correspondences: Bladder, kidneys and adrenal glands, hips, and spleen.

Mind: Soothing Jade assists in integrating the mind with the body, stabilizing the personality. It releases obsessive and negative thoughts and simplifies the organization of tasks.

Emotions: Jade facilitates healing the trauma of past grief, which has been suppressed and has become locked within the emotional energy field. It also calms irritability and brings inner peace.

Jade is one of the oldest-known healing stones of China.

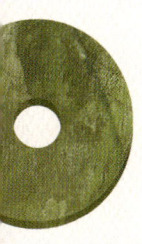

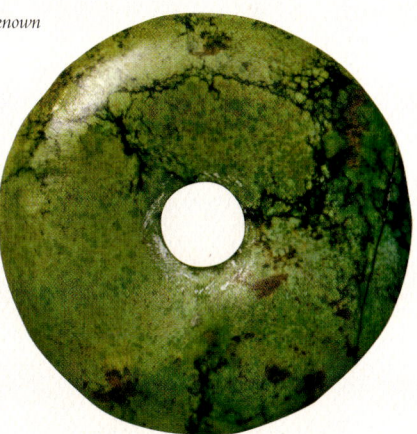

Spirit: This crystal traditionally signifies wholeness and peace. It encourages becoming who you really are, and assists you in recognizing yourself as a spiritual being. Meditate with Jade and clearly picture any positive changes that you wish to put in place, to offset the negative expectations that surround you.

Curious fact: Ancient Chinese royalty were often interred in intricately constructed suits of jade and gold armour, which were believed to confer protection and immortality.

Did you know? Jade has long been a symbol of purity and serenity. Much prized in the East, it signifies wisdom garnered in tranquillity.

Hot tip: Wear or carry this stone over the centre of your upper chest to stimulate your physical and psychic immune system, and place it on your forehead to bring you insightful dreams. Jade is also believed to be particularly protective for lone travellers.

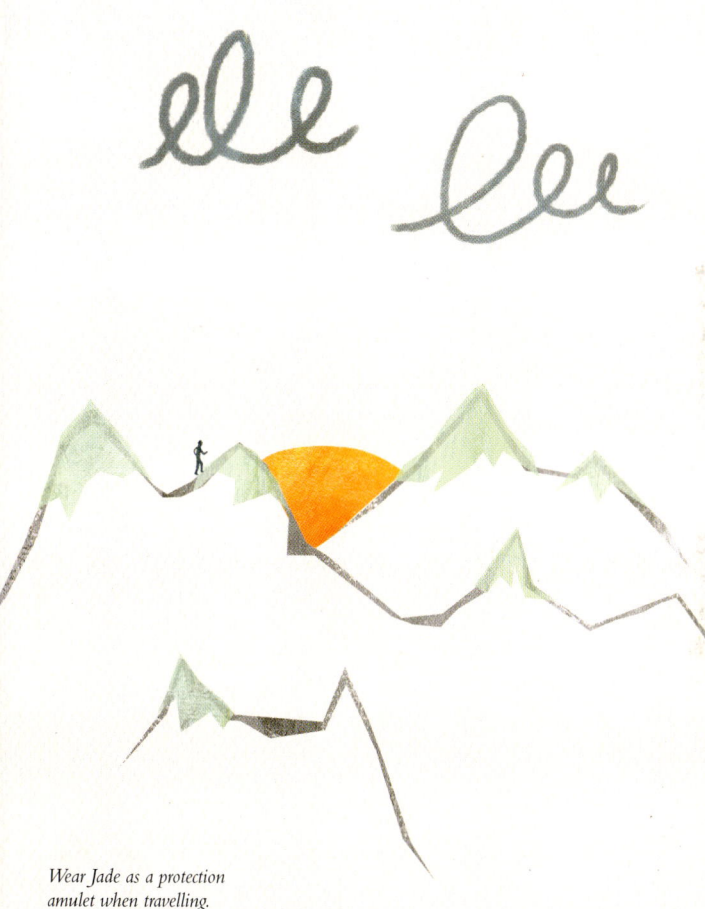

Wear Jade as a protection amulet when travelling.

Jade 45

Red Jasper: Vitality

Red Jasper is a powerful and energetic stone. Carrying this crystal with you livens up your life considerably, as it's something of a party animal, and traditionally was said to prolong sexual pleasure.

Known as the "stone of perpetual protection", in ancient times Red Jasper was very popular for amulets. In 15th-century German high magic, it acted against "offensive imaginings" and in the 16th century it expelled "noxious phantasms". It is useful if you are overwhelmed by nightmares or beset by evil entities, and is the stone of the Apostle Peter and the Archangel Haniel, ruling over the Angelic Principalities.

> *Red Jasper brings good luck to child and man [and] drives away all evil things, to thee and thine protection brings.*
> *Johann Wolfgang von Goethe (1749–1832),*
> *German writer and statesman*

Body: Red Jasper is the go-to stone whenever you need extra energy or stamina. This is a stone of health, traditionally strengthening and detoxifying the circulatory system and the blood and liver. It appears in the very earliest crystal-healing recipes. It is helpful for prolonged convalescence, speeding up recovery time. Traditionally Red Jasper increases fertility and creativity, overcoming impotence at any level.

Physiological correspondences: Circulation, digestion, sexual function, the reproductive organs, liver; mineral assimilation.

Mind: Stimulating the imagination, Red Jasper helps you to "think on your feet". It brings you the courage to get to grips with problems assertively before they become too big, and to see projects through. This stone heightens organizational abilities, helping you transform ideas into action. When placed under your pillow, it assists dream recall.

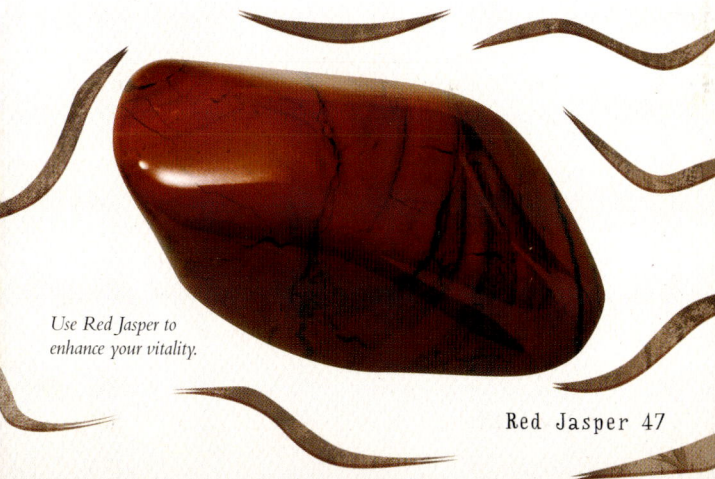

Use Red Jasper to enhance your vitality.

Emotions: Red Jasper encourages you to be honest with yourself. It makes an excellent "worry bead", calming the emotions when gently stroked. However, it can also inflame the passions.

Spirit: This crystal keeps your feet on the ground and offers protection to your spirit. It cleans and stabilizes the aura, and strengthens your energetic boundaries. At the same time it reminds us all to help each other.

Curious fact: In Egyptian times Red Jasper was associated with the menstrual blood of the goddess Isis, and was used to assist pregnant woman and to increase lactation following childbirth.

Did you know? In the language of gemstones, Red Jasper symbolizes courage and wisdom. In scrying – using crystals to foresee the future – it signifies that your love is reciprocated.

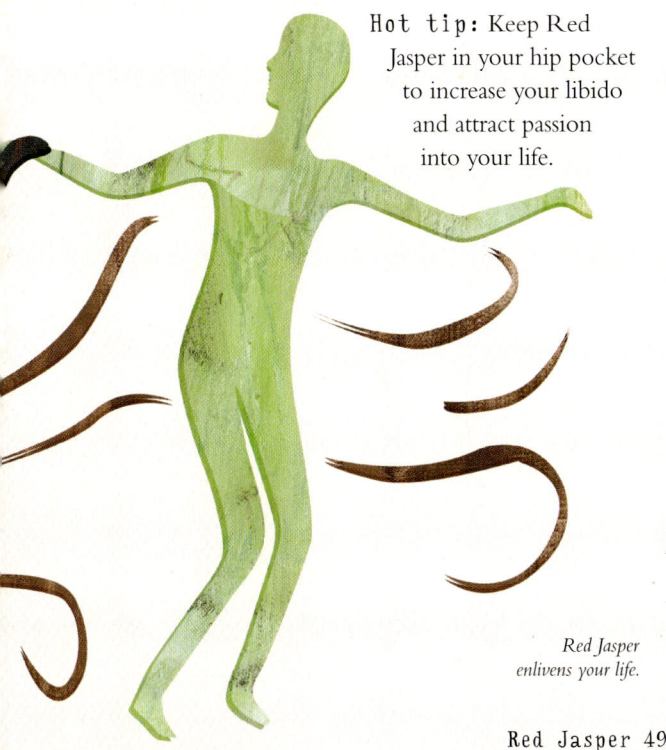

Hot tip: Keep Red Jasper in your hip pocket to increase your libido and attract passion into your life.

Red Jasper enlivens your life.

Eye of the Storm (Judy's Jasper): Stability

Eye of the Storm is a combination of Agate and Jasper. Holding this stone is like standing in the eye of a hurricane: everything is swirling around you, but you are in the still centre. You can hunker down and be protected, or you can rise up and take the bigger view.

This crystal reminds you that the picture is fluid and can change, depending on actions taken and decisions made; in this space, solutions become apparent. The stone acts as a life-support system for you and the planet – the world becomes lighter, brighter, and more balanced, with this stone in your pocket.

> *The cyclone derives its power from a calm centre.*
> *So does a person.*
> *Norman Vincent Peale (1898–1993),*
> *visionary writer*

Body: This stone is an excellent stress-reliever that switches off the body's "fight or flight" response when it feels threatened. It contains dynamic raw energy on which to draw, and some claim it encourages the growth of healthy new cells.

Promoting a natural detox on all levels, Eye of the Storm releases pressure on the kidneys and balances the organs of the body.

Physiological correspondences: Adrenals, kidneys, pancreas, spleen, eyes; blood pressure, cellular walls.

Mind: This crystal shows you the bigger picture, so that you can make fully informed decisions and recognize the potential that is opening up to you. It also shows where you may have exaggerated apparent problems to a level where you have been so obsessed by them that you have missed the essence of the matter. For example, losing a job could turn out to be the best thing that has happened to you, as it may open the way for the perfect job to materialize.

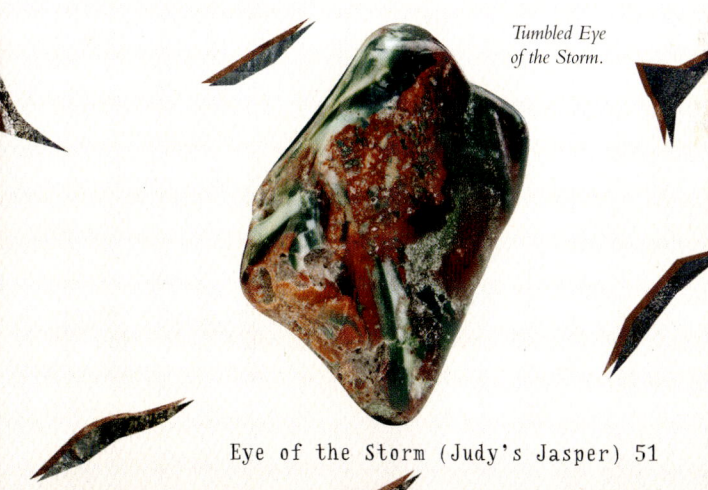

Tumbled Eye of the Storm.

Emotions: This stone reprogrammes any sense of loss or lack into positive abundance.

Spirit: Eye of the Storm takes you back to your spiritual roots – what the ancient Egyptians called "Zep Tepi", or the first time, an age when humanity and nature were in harmony together, as were body and soul.

Curious fact: This crystal is currently being trialled as a support system following chemotherapy, because it sustains during serious illness.

Did you know? "Judy's Jasper" was named after Judy Hall by experienced crystal worker John van Rees. "Eye of the Storm" is the name given to it by Judy herself, as she feels this more properly reflects its true properties.

Hot tip: Wear this stone constantly when you are under any kind of stress.

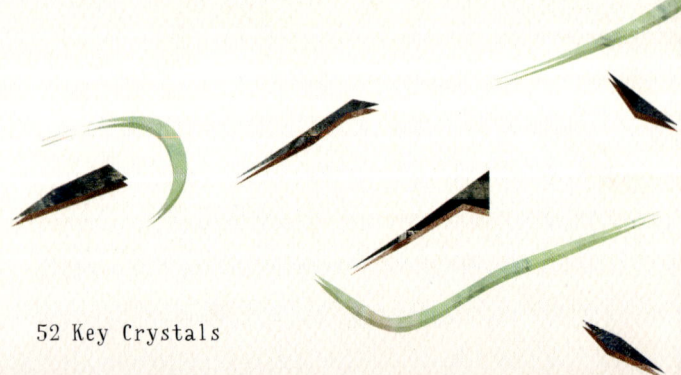

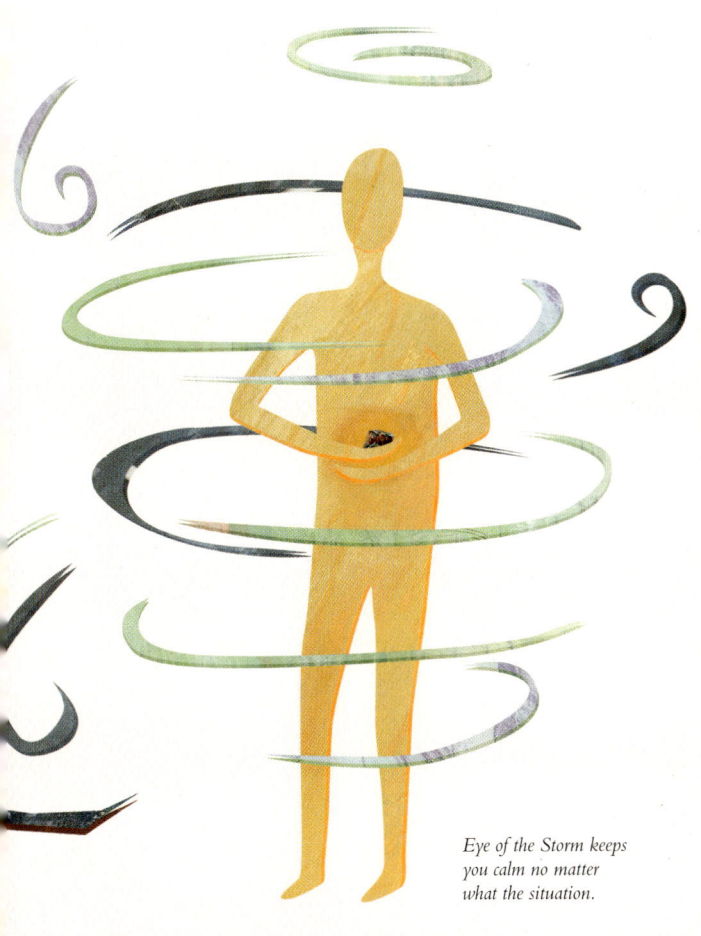

*Eye of the Storm keeps
you calm no matter
what the situation.*

Eye of the Storm (Judy's Jasper) 53

Goldstone: Wealth

Sold as "the money stone", shiny, gem-like Goldstone is artificially created from glass and copper. It helps you perform financial alchemy and has traditionally been used to attract wealth of all kinds.

The best-quality stone is found at the heart of the mass: when cracked open and smoothed to reveal its beauty, it symbolizes the inner processes that must occur before transmutation can manifest.

There is much debate in the crystal-healing world as to whether or not Goldstone is a healing stone: some people come out strongly in its favour, whereas others say it has little value. But it has acquired a healing reputation by virtue of long use and its component materials – copper being a powerful healing mineral. So try the stone and make up your own mind.

Not what we have but what we enjoy
constitutes our abundance.
Epicurus (341–270BCE),
Greek philosopher

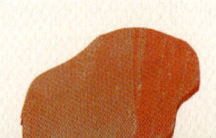

Body: Goldstone is reported to detoxify the body. With its copper content, it is helpful for easing arthritic pain and strengthening bones. And its sparkiness acts as an antidote for depression.

Physiological correspondences: Circulatory system.

Mind: Goldstone teaches that what your mind conceives, it achieves – so you had better think positively!

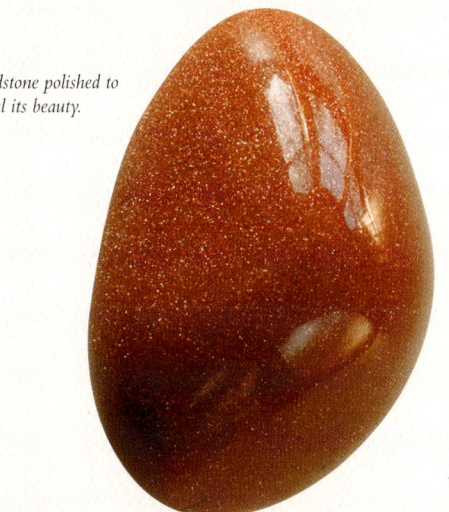

Goldstone polished to reveal its beauty.

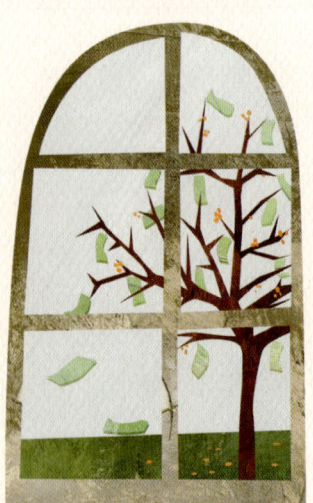

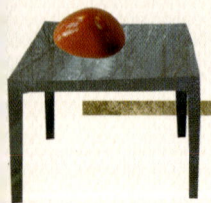

Place your Goldstone in the Wealth Corner.

56 Key Crystals

Emotions: This crystal helps you to stay calm and stabilizes your emotions.

Spirit: Goldstone lifts the spirits, but its real benefits lie elsewhere.

Curious fact: Goldstone was created by alchemists as they sought to make gold. An Italian monastic order was among those who made it, to a jealously guarded secret recipe, as were the Miotti glass-making family in 17th-century Venice. Goldstone was especially prized by the Chinese, who called it jinxing boli, meaning "gold star glass". During its manufacture, the molten glass has to be kept at a specific temperature until the mineral salts have crystallized out into their spectacular colours.

Did you know? Abundance is more than having money; it is an attitude of mind. A strong inner sense of abundant wellbeing opens up infinite possibilities. Being abundant means living in a deeply enriched way – physically, mentally, emotionally, and spiritually. It is founded upon valuing yourself and your life, exactly as you are right now.

Hot tip: Place Goldstone in the wealth corner of your house – the furthest back left-hand corner from the front door – to bring you prosperity.

Green Aventurine: Success

Green Aventurine is a stone of prosperity
and one of the premier crystals for
attracting luck, abundance, and success.
It reinforces leadership qualities and
decisiveness, but also teaches that you
do not have to be successful in the eyes
of the world to enjoy a fulfilling life.

This stone shows you that "failure" is not a mistake, but
rather part of the learning process – it helps you to value
what you have, and encourages you to try again, setting
achievable goals instead of indulging in pipe dreams.

Green Aventurine assists you to recognize (and
overcome) any inner feelings of lack, or "poverty
consciousness", that may be holding you back. This
supportive stone releases your reliance on other people,
showing you that You Can Do It. If you need to step
outside your comfort zone, Green Aventurine increases
your confidence and helps you to become your true self.

Shall life succeed in that it seems to fail:
What I aspired to be,
And was not, comforts me.
Robert Browning (1812–80),
English poet and playwright

Body: Green Aventurine promotes a feeling of wellbeing. It also regulates growth from birth to the age of seven years.

Physiological correspondences: Spleen, eyes, lungs, heart, skin, adrenals, sinuses, muscular and urogenital systems, thymus, metabolic processes, nervous system, connective tissue.

Mind: One of the stones of creativity, Green Aventurine stabilizes your state of mind. It stimulates perception and helps you to assess alternatives and possibilities, especially those presented by other people.

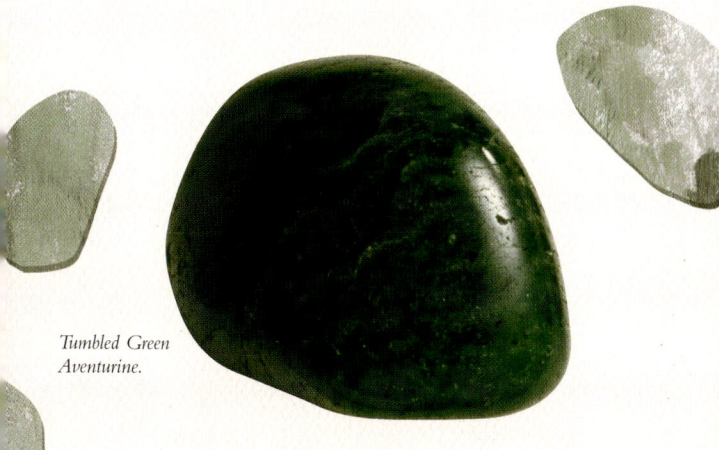

Tumbled Green Aventurine.

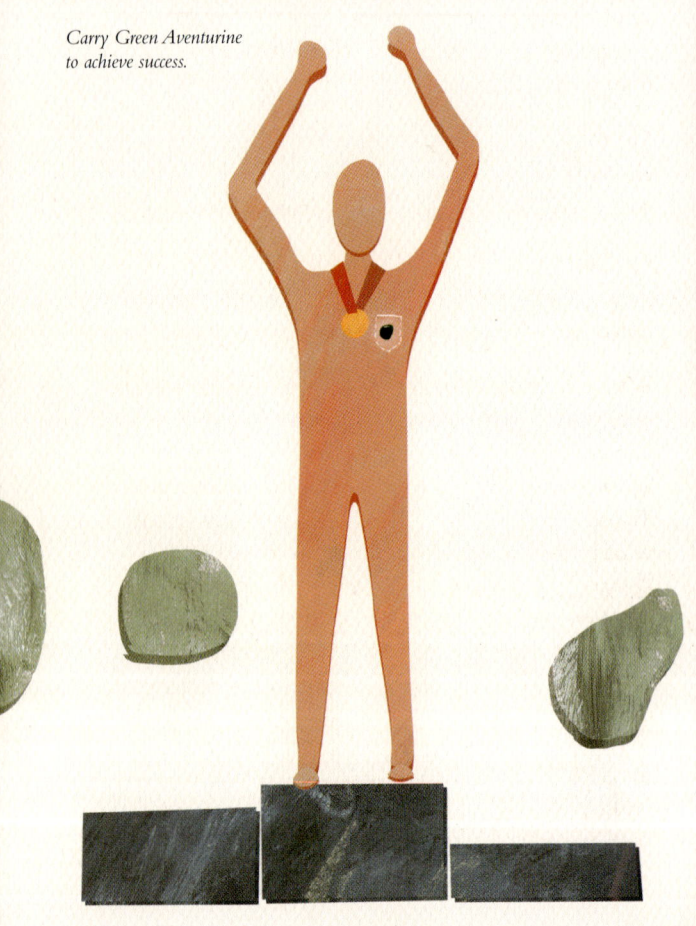

*Carry Green Aventurine
to achieve success.*

60 Key Crystals

Emotions: This crystal calms anger and irritation. It also supports emotional recovery and helps you to live from your heart.

Spirit: Green Aventurine activates and protects the heart chakra. It keeps the psychic vampires (people who suck out your energy and leave you feeling drained) away, too!

Curious fact: Green Aventurine is named from the Italian *all'avventura*, meaning "by chance", because it is usually found by accident.

Did you know? An opaque form of Quartz or Feldspar with sparkly Pyrite inclusions, Green Aventurine was well known in the ancient world, and there are many statues and amulets made of this glittering stone in museums. Translation problems make it difficult to assess exactly what properties were traditionally attributed to it. "Smargos" – green stone – is often translated as Emerald, but these were rare. It could be Green Quartz, Green Aventurine, or Jade. The "emerald" mentioned in connection with the biblical Breastplate of the High Priest is more likely to have been Green Aventurine.

Hot tip: Keep Green Aventurine in your left-hand breast-pocket or wear it constantly, so that you stand in your own power and attract success to you.

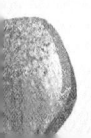
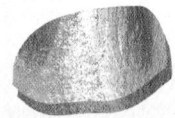

Rose Quartz:
Love and relationships

This peaceful crystal is known as the "Stone of Unconditional Love" and it transforms relationships with yourself and others, creating love and harmony.

Rose Quartz is also a wonderful stone to use during a midlife crisis or in traumatic circumstances. It helps you take an objective look at a situation without being emotionally overwhelmed. This beautiful stone teaches you how to love and accept yourself, forgiving the past and living from your heart. If you feel disempowered or unloved, hold Rose Quartz and remind yourself of a time when you felt totally positive, potent, loved, and accepted – the crystal will bring that feeling into the present moment.

Kindness in words creates confidence.
Kindness in thinking creates profoundness.
Kindness in giving creates love.
Lao Tzu (flourished 6th century BCE),
Chinese philosopher

Body: This gentle stone harmonizes the brain, aligning and opening neural pathways. When placed over the centre of your chest, it calms an asthma attack or other breathing difficulties. It is also helpful for dissolving the psychosomatic causes of dis-ease.

Physiological correspondences: Heart, blood, circulation, thymus, lungs, adrenals, skin, brainstem, reproductive and lymphatic systems.

Mind: Rose Quartz supports your positive affirmations. Wearing the stone will remind you of your intention.

Rose Quartz shaped into a love-heart.

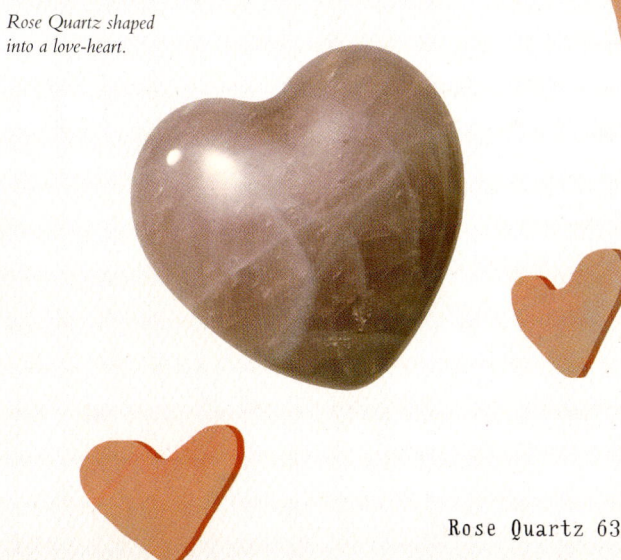

Emotions: This crystal is an emotional healer par excellence. It releases and transmutes previously blocked emotions and dissolves guilt and bitterness. It is the perfect stone for healing a broken heart.

Spirit: Rose Quartz opens the heart chakra and connects you to a never-ending supply of unconditional love and compassion. It also opens the third eye (the "eye of insight" associated with the brow chakra in the centre of the forehead), offering you metaphysical gifts such as clairvoyance and telepathy.

Curious fact: Although Rose Quartz has been known as the Stone of Unconditional Love for many years, there are no records of its use in ancient times, and no talismans have been found carved from this beautiful stone.

Did you know? In the Middle Ages, Rose Quartz was regarded as a precious gemstone in Bohemia, and it decorated the St Wenceslas Chapel in Prague. Like King Arthur in England, Wenceslas – patron saint of the Czech Republic – is said to sleep with his knights under a mountain and will awaken to aid his country at its time of greatest need.

Hot tip: If you want to attract more love into your life, place a large Rose Quartz beside your bed.

Keep Rose Quartz by your bed to attract harmonious love.

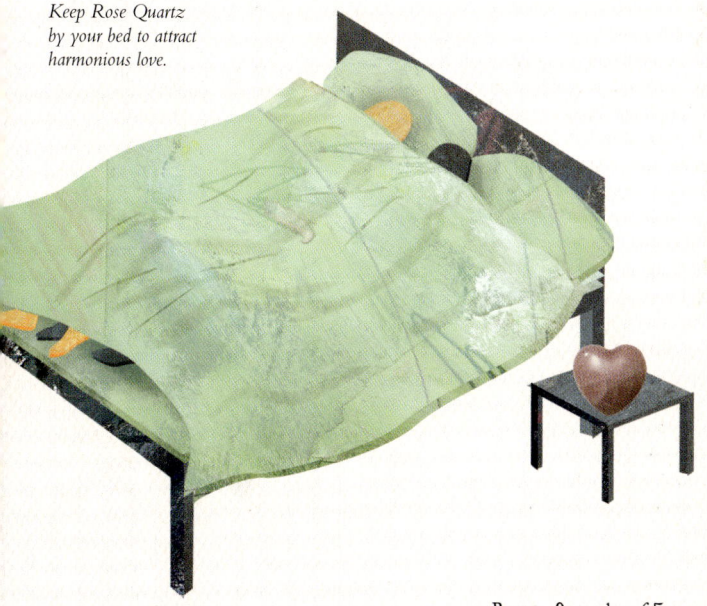

Citrine: Career

Citrine is a happy, generous stone. It
stimulates living in the moment rather
than in your dreams. This crystal gives
you the energy to manifest your own
reality. Demonstrating the old adage that
"like follows like", it encourages you to
notice with gratitude all the small joys
of everyday life, and suggests that you
share what you have and take pleasure
in the giving.

Citrine helps you to succeed in your chosen career as it
harmonizes your purpose to your everyday life and helps
you to find joy in all you do. This crystal also teaches that
when you do what you love, success follows. With Citrine
in your pocket, you will fulfil your dreams because you
recognize that the universe – and your soul – wants you
to succeed.

*There is no passion to be found in playing small – in
settling for a life that is less than you are capable of living.
Nelson Mandela (1918–2013), South African
nationalist and politician*

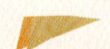

Body: Citrine is a useful stone for energizing and recharging yourself. It has a warming effect and fortifies the nerves.

Physiological correspondences: Detoxification, circulation and energy systems; thymus, thyroid, spleen, pancreas, kidneys, bladder, female reproductive system.

Mind: Citrine promotes inner calm, so that wisdom can emerge. It enhances your concentration, assisting you in digesting information, analysing situations, and steering them in a positive direction. It also encourages individuality. This crystal strengthens your motivation, activates your creativity, and encourages self-expression. It makes you less sensitive to criticism, so that you respond constructively. With this stone you will develop a positive attitude and

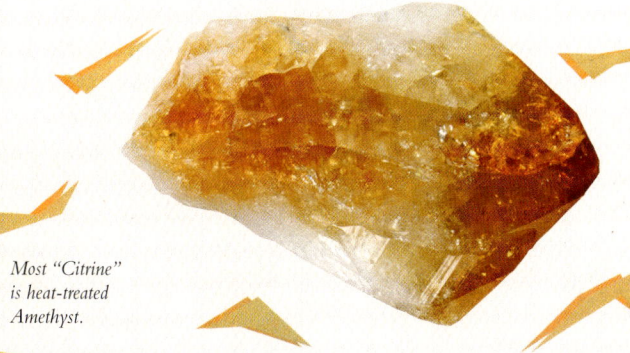

*Most "Citrine"
is heat-treated
Amethyst.*

look forward optimistically; it encourages the enjoyment of new experiences, and exploration of every possible avenue until you find the best solution. Wearing a Citrine pendant overcomes difficulties in verbalizing thoughts and feelings.

Emotions: This crystal raises your self-esteem and self-confidence. It is excellent for overcoming depression, fears, and phobias. By helping you to overcome destructive tendencies, it brings joy to your life. If what you do never seems good enough, keep Citrine with you at all times.

Spirit: This stone will bring joy to your soul.

Curious fact: The same mineral (iron) colours natural Citrine, red Haematite, brown Bronzite, and purple Amethyst. Most bright-yellow or brownish Citrines are actually heat-treated Amethyst.

Did you know? Citrine is known as the "Merchant Stone", because it was traditionally kept in cash boxes to attract money and success.

Hot tip: This stone knows that what your mind conceives, it achieves. So focus on what you want to attract right now, put that intention into the crystal, then let it go.

Citrine gives you confidence when speaking in public.

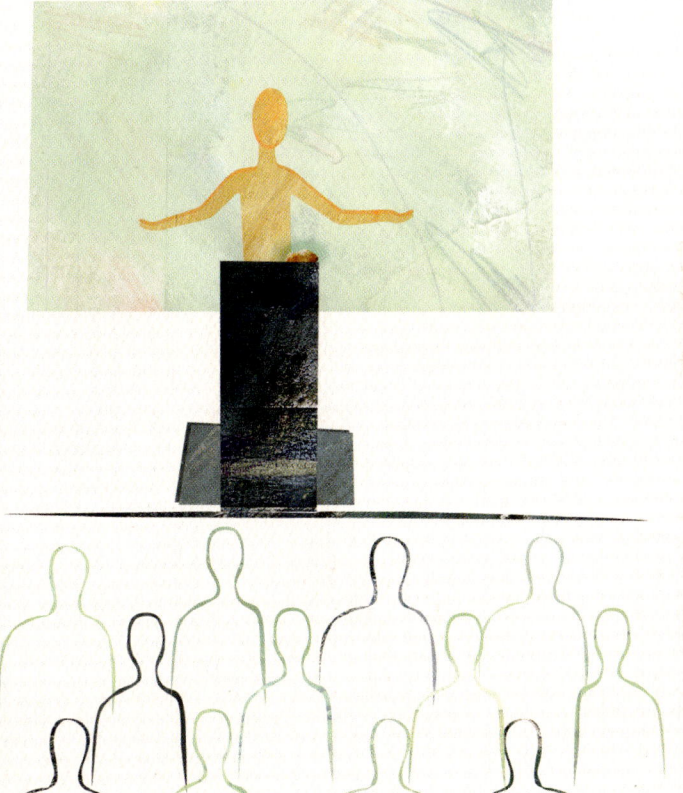

Citrine 69

Black Tourmaline: Protection

Black Tourmaline is invaluable for
electro-sensitive people, who are overwhelmed
by geopathic or electromagnetic stress
or radiation (namely the subtle but
detectable electromagnetic field or
vibrational conflicts given off by power
lines and electrical equipment). Place
this crystal around your home to create
a protective space that blocks out
negativity or toxic energy of any kind; or
attach it to a phone, tablet, or computer.
It is also a powerful personal protection
stone against jealousy or ill-wishing.

Connecting with the base chakra, Black Tourmaline
grounds energy and increases physical vitality, dispersing
tension and stress. It has iron in it, but due to its inner
structure, it traps negative energy rather than amplifying
it, as iron-based stones are prone to do.

> *This Tourmaline will not only attract ashes from burning*
> *coals, but will also repel them again, in an amusing way...*
> *as if they were appearing to writhe themselves by force*
> *into the stone, they, in a little time, spring from it again.*
> *Theophrastus (c.381–287BCE),* On Stones

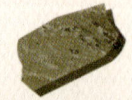

Body: Black Tourmaline increases wellbeing, by screening out toxic or negative energies so that they cannot affect you. It harmonizes the brain and re-patterns neural-pathway malfunctions. It also stimulates the immune system and the thyroid. Hold this crystal for pain relief and to relieve arthritic swelling.

Physiological correspondences: Immune system, spinal column, motor function, lungs; detoxification.

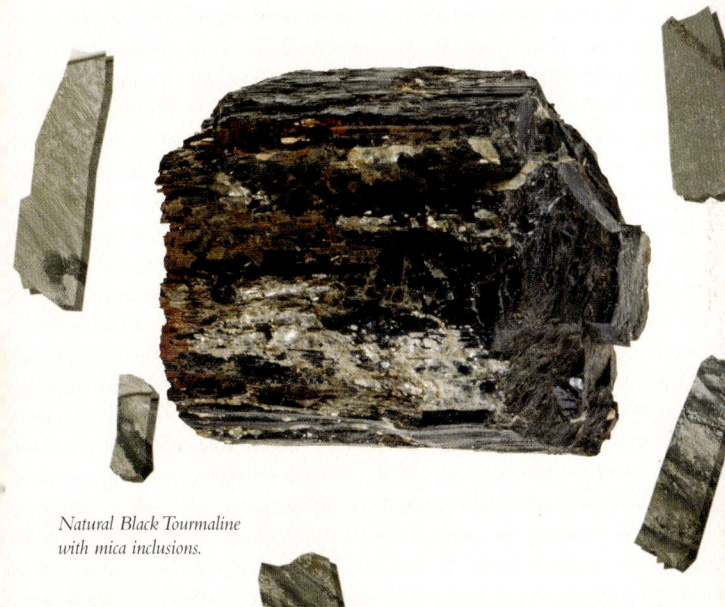

Natural Black Tourmaline with mica inclusions.

Mind: With its ability to clear negative thoughts, Black Tourmaline promotes a laid-back attitude and clear, rational thought processes. It encourages a positive approach, no matter what the circumstances. This is a great stone for altruism and practical creativity. Black Tourmaline also helps you to recognize that, by holding on to negative thoughts or toxic emotions, you attack yourself from within.

Black Tourmaline creates powerful protection.

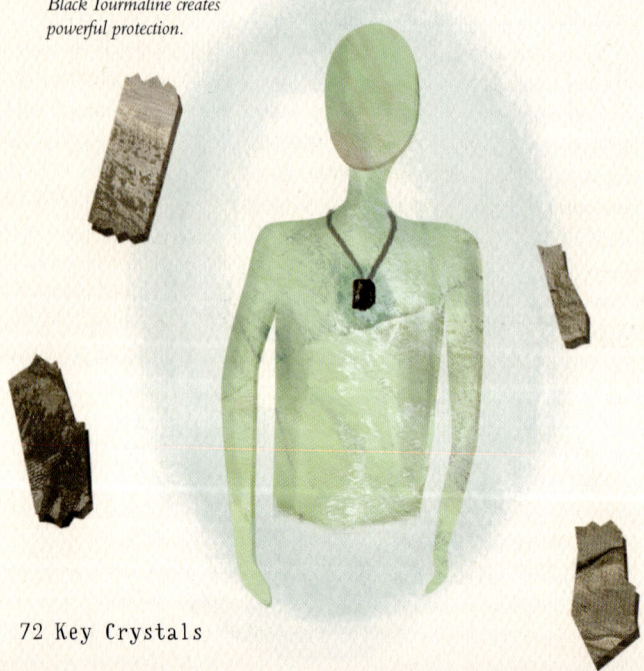

Emotions: This crystal assists you in understanding yourself and others. It takes you deep into yourself, to banish fear and find self-confidence. It overcomes the feeling of being a victim and encourages compassion, tolerance, and positivity.

Spirit: Black Tourmaline grounds and protects the soul.

Curious fact: Burmese Black Tourmaline was traditionally sent to China, for cutting into buttons for mandarins' hats.

Did you know? Black Tourmaline is both piezoelectric and pyroelectric – that is, it generates electricity through pressure and through heat, such as the sun. It also absorbs light, which it later releases. Due to its electrostatic properties of attraction and repulsion, it was named the "ash-drawer" – a property that, apparently, was discovered accidentally by some Dutch children when playing with this stone. Old Dutchmen traditionally used it to draw the ashes out of their pipe.

Hot tip: Wear Black Tourmaline around your neck to help prevent you from inadvertently upsetting someone.

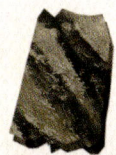

Turquoise: Totem

Turquoise is a totem for good health and is the perfect protection stone, having long been used for amulets. It contains traces of iron, which is noted for its protective qualities.

A turquoise given by a loving hand carries
with it happiness and good fortune.
Arab proverb

Body: Losing its colour in the presence of illness, Turquoise strengthens the immune system and the subtle meridians of the body. This stone is helpful for physical or mental exhaustion. It encourages tissue regeneration and the assimilation of nutrients. In early crystal lore, drinking Turquoise-infused water alleviated urine retention. This crystal contains copper, long prized for its anti-inflammatory properties. In crystal healing it is a pain-reliever and assists cramp, arthritis, and similar dis-eases. Turquoise has also been prescribed for sore throats for thousands of years: it contains phosphoric acid, which, if given in a large dose, would sear the throat, but when used homeopathically as a crystal, the vibration from Turquoise soothes the throat.

Physiological correspondences: Throat, eyes, tissues, immune system; energy meridians, assimilation of nutrients, pain receptors.

Mind: Psychologically Turquoise is a strengthening stone, and dissolves self-sabotage or feelings of victimhood. It instils inner calm, while helping you to remain alert. It also assists creative expression.

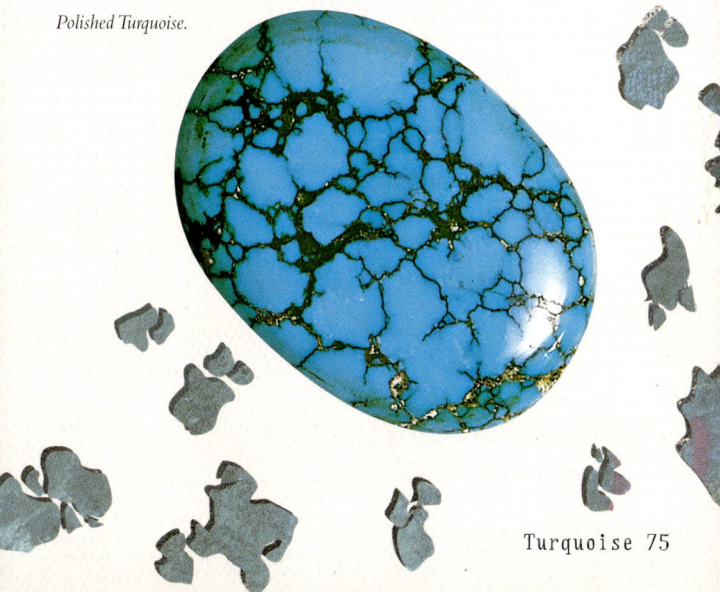

Polished Turquoise.

Emotions: This crystal stabilizes mood swings and brings inner peace. It lifts the depression caused by adverse circumstances.

Spirit: Turquoise promotes spiritual attunement and enhances communication with the physical and spiritual worlds. When placed on the third eye in the centre of the forehead, it increases intuition and facilitates meditation.

Curious fact: According to Pueblo legend, Turquoise stole its colour from the sky, so it symbolizes humanity's cosmic origins.

Did you know? Use of this crystal goes way back into prehistory, and it has long been regarded as a powerful protector against the evil eye. Turquoise amulets and statuettes have been found in Egyptian and Greco-Roman tombs, and the stone was sacred to the Egyptian goddess Hathor, the Roman goddess Venus, and Aphrodite in Greece – the goddess of love, sex, beauty, and fertility. Turquoise was also considered sacred by the Aztecs and

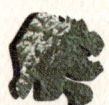

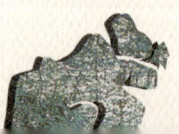

the Native Americans. It was brought back to Europe by the crusaders. In the East, horses' bridles were set with Turquoise to ensure that no accidents befell the rider; the stone was believed to draw into itself any harm directed towards the wearer.

`Hot tip:` Programme your Turquoise to keep you safe from harm, and wear it constantly around your wrist or at your throat.

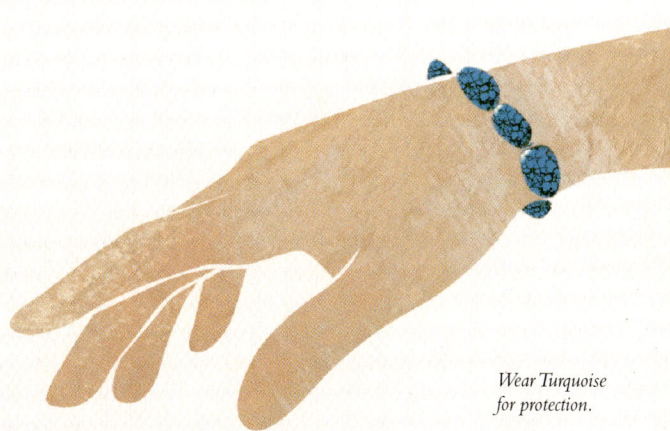

Wear Turquoise for protection.

Amethyst: Meditation

Amethyst is an excellent aid to meditation, because it turns your thoughts away from the mundane and towards tranquillity and deeper understanding. It can help you to recall and interpret your dreams and, when placed over the third eye, it aids visualization.

In the attitude of silence the soul finds the path in a clearer light, and what is elusive and deceptive resolves itself into crystal clearness.
Mahatma Gandhi (1869–1948), Indian nationalist and politician

Body: Amethyst boosts the endocrine system – the collection of glands that secrete hormones into the circulation. It also assists the transmission of neural signals through the brain. When placed under your pillow, this crystal is helpful if you suffer from insomnia caused by an overactive mind, and is also used to protect against recurrent nightmares. In ancient times Amethyst was bound to the forehead to cure a headache. Today crystal workers use this stone to draw off physical or psychological pain and to calm anxiety. It facilitates multi-dimensional cellular healing.

Physiological correspondences: Cellular and metabolic processes, endocrine function and hormone regulation, neural transmission, and brain harmonization; immune system, blood, skin, respiration, digestive tract, skin, psychosomatic disorders.

Mind: Amethyst stills the mind and promotes mindfulness. It helps you to feel more focused and less scattered, assisting the decision-making process. The crystal is a natural tranquillizer and excellent for counteracting mental stress.

Emotions: This stone is helpful for understanding the deeper causes that lie behind addictions and offers support during withdrawal from substance abuse. It calms anxiety and lifts depression.

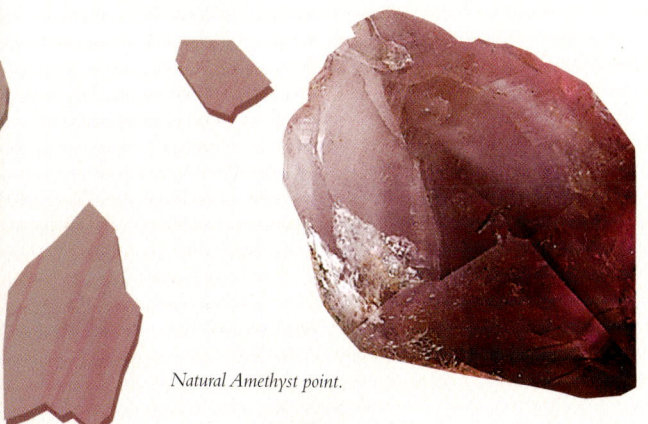

Natural Amethyst point.

*Amethyst instils
peace of mind.*

80 Key Crystals

Spirit: Amethyst is one of the most spiritual stones and creates a safe, sacred space for meditation. When placed above the head, it activates the higher chakras and facilitates enlightenment.

Curious fact: The name "Amethyst" literally means "not drunk" – and this crystal has been worn as a talisman against drunkenness for millennia.

Did you know? According to myth, the god of wine, Bacchus, was offended by Diana, the huntress. In a fit of pique, he declared that the first person he met in the forest would be eaten by his tiger. A beautiful maiden called Amethyst met the tiger. When she called on the goddess to save her, Diana turned her into a sparkling white crystal. Feeling contrite, Bacchus poured wine over the crystal, turning it purple.

Hot tip: Lie down, then place one Amethyst point above your head facing down, and one on your third eye in the middle of your forehead, also pointing down. Close your eyes and feel the peace radiating through your body.

Selenite: Spirituality

Translucent Selenite has a very fine vibration, opening the higher crown chakras to access angelic consciousness and spiritual guidance. It is one of the most powerful crystals for anchoring a new vibration on Earth.

Selenite has long been regarded as "frozen divine light". It brings this divine light into anything it touches, raising the energetic frequency of the human body and of the planet. This stone is a powerful transmutor for emotional energy, helping to release core toxic feelings that lie behind psychosomatic illnesses and emotional blockages. This creates the space for a vibrational uplift, rather like installing a new computer program. This uplift is often referred to as "ascension".

> *The Universe consists of frozen light.*
> *David Bohm (1917–92), American scientist*

Body: Selenite's most profound healing occurs at an energetic rather than a physical level, although it aligns the spinal column and promotes flexibility. Crystal workers use selenite to ameliorate the detrimental effects of dental amalgam (an alloy of mercury and other metals) and free radicals.

Physiological correspondences: Spinal column, joints, breasts, nerves; puberty, the menopause.

Mind: Selenite brings clarity to your mind. It clears confusion and facilitates seeing the deeper picture. Meditating with this crystal brings about a conscious understanding of what has been occurring at the subconscious level. It assists judgement and insight.

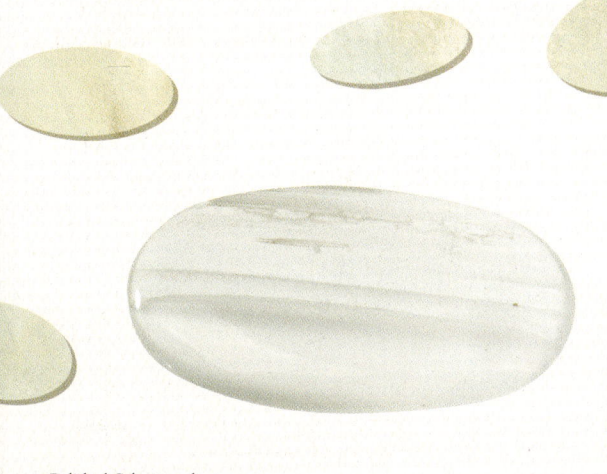

Polished Selenite palmstone.

Emotions: This stone is an emotional stabilizer, calming mood swings.

Spirit: When you hold Selenite, you are connected to the higher realms. This stone stimulates the high-vibration chakras, opening your psychic abilities. It pinpoints issues from previous lives, and shows you how they can best be resolved.

Curious fact: The 13th-century Lapidary of King Alphonso X the Learned of Spain (a lapidary being a text about the properties of precious and semi-precious stones) tells us that this stone can only be found at night by the light of the full moon. The Lapidary recommends Selenite as a cure for epilepsy – a belief brought forward from ancient times.

Did you know? This crystal has long been viewed as representing the interface between the material and the divine worlds. Known as "crystalline divine light", Selenite was sacred to the Greek moon goddess Selene, and to the even more ancient Mesopotamian god Ninurta (Saturn in Roman belief).

Hot tip: Place Selenite above your head to connect you to the highest possible spiritual forces.

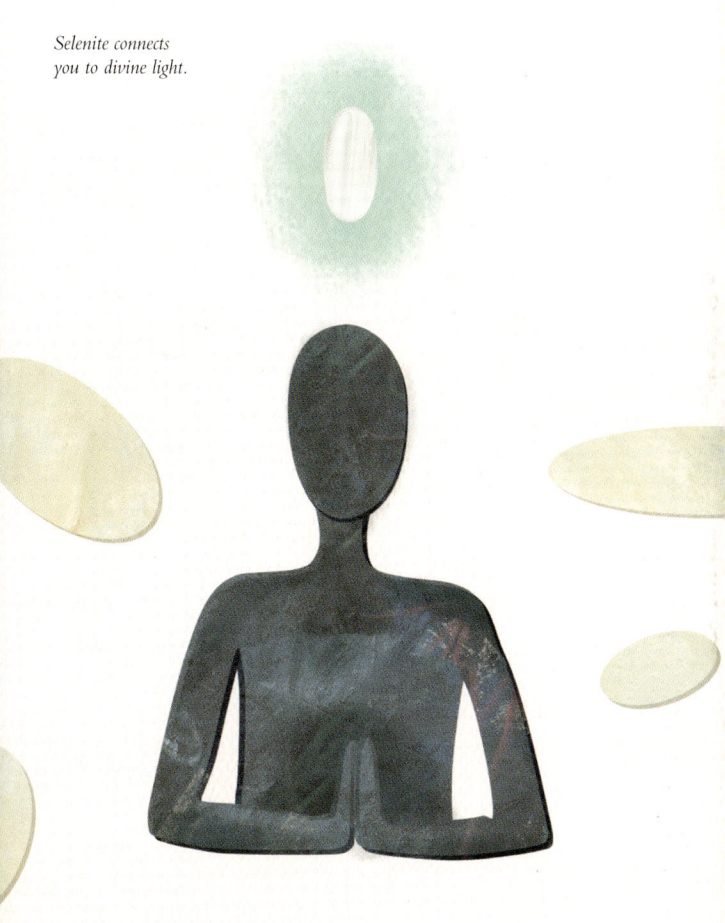

*Selenite connects
you to divine light.*

Selenite 85

Quartz: Safe, sacred space

A master healer, Quartz is the most abundant crystal on the planet and was traditionally regarded as a medicine stone of great power throughout the ancient and not-so-ancient worlds.

It works at a vibrational level, attuned to the specific energy requirements of the person who needs healing or who undertakes spiritual work. It takes the energy to the most perfect state possible, going back to the time before any dis-ease set in. This deep soul-cleanser removes the seeds of karmic dis-ease (that is, disease resulting from your own actions), detoxifies the emotional field, and clarifies the mind.

The Roman geographer Pliny bemoans the fact that many pieces of Quartz are impaired by defects such as "rough solder-like excrescences", occlusions of water, cloudy or "salt-spots", bright red rust, and internal fibres – all prized by crystal workers today for the properties they add to the underlying crystal.
Judy Hall, 101 Power Crystals

Body: Quartz brings the body into balance, treating any condition, and among its benefits are the regeneration of

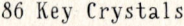

cells and the regulation of blood pressure. This stone is composed of silica, which is essential for the maintenance of healthy, well-oxygenated cells and is one of the building blocks of the immune system.

Physiological correspondences: All the systems and organs of the physical and subtle bodies; mineral assimilation.

Mind: This crystal brings clarity and focus to the mind, unlocking stored memories.

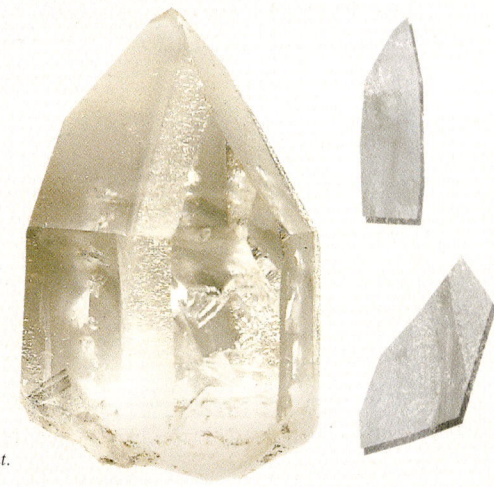

Natural Quartz point.

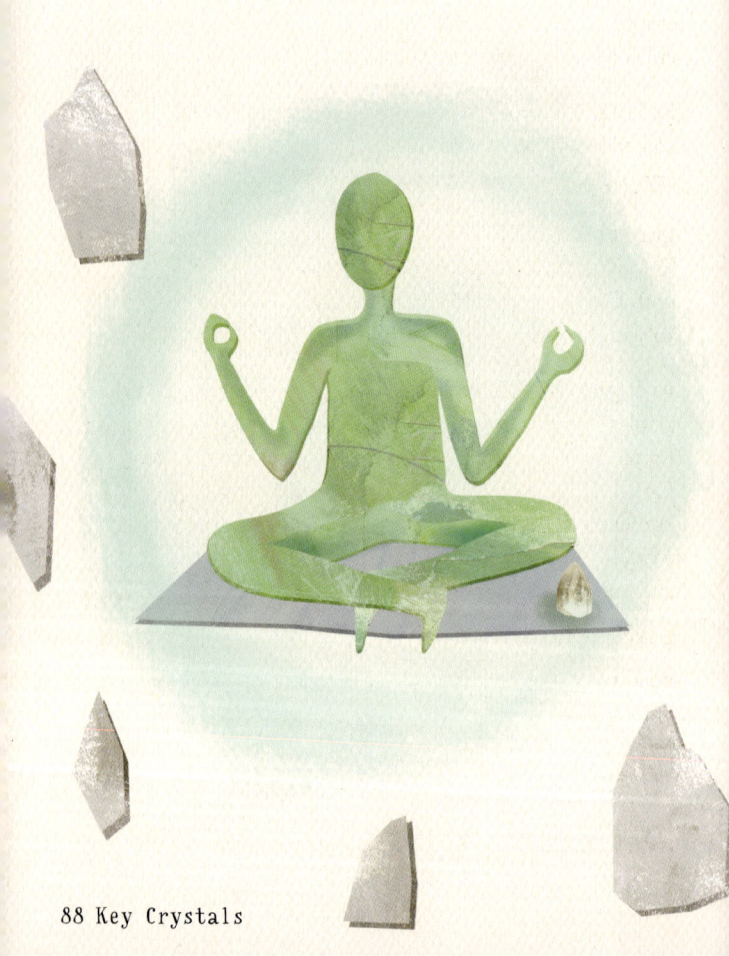

88 Key Crystals

Emotions: Quartz can facilitate a powerful, yet gentle emotional detox, clearing away detritus from the past and enhancing positive emotions.

Spirit: This stone is a consciousness-raiser. With their ability to store information, like a natural computer, Quartz crystals are a spiritual library waiting to be read.

Curious fact: A 5th-century BCE Greek priest, Onomacritus, tells us that anyone entering a temple with Quartz in their hand is certain to have their prayers answered, as the gods cannot resist its power.

Did you know? Native Americans placed Quartz in the cradles of newborn infants to make a connection to the Earth. They called this stone "the brain cells of Mother Earth". Its piezoelectric qualities mean that it can generate, conserve, and pass on energy. Without Quartz, computers wouldn't run, early radios would not have come into being, and energy could not be transmitted around energy grids.

Hot tip: Place a large Quartz crystal wherever you need to create a safe, sacred space in which to expand your spirituality.

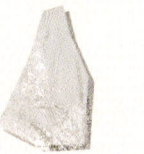

Quartz harmonizes brainwaves and prepares you for meditation.

Smoky Quartz:
Everyday living

Smoky Quartz is one of the premier grounding
and anchoring stones. Strongly protective
and detoxifying, it is a highly versatile
healer, which can reverse the effects
of electromagnetic pollution, geopathic
stress, and negative energies generally.

Place this crystal at your feet, or on the base of your spine,
to strengthen your core stability. Position it pointing
outwards to draw off negative energies; pointing inwards
to energize the body. The stone is excellent for earth-
healing and for space-clearing your home.

> *Justice shines in very smoky homes, and honours*
> *the righteous; but the gold-spangled mansions where the*
> *hands are unclean she leaves with eyes averted.*
> *Aeschylus (c.525–456BCE), Agamemnon, l.773*

Body: Smoky Quartz is particularly effective for ailments
of the abdomen, hips, and legs. It provides pain relief and
dissolves cramp. Traditionally it strengthens the back and
fortifies the nerves. It also works on the kidneys and other
organs of elimination to remove toxins from the body.

Physiological correspondences: Abdomen, legs, feet, muscles; nervous, reproductive, and elimination systems; the assimilation of minerals, fluid regulation, detoxification.

Mind: A superb antidote to stress, Smoky Quartz helps you to tolerate difficult times with equanimity, fortifying your resolve. If your survival instincts are low or you feel depleted of energy, the psychological strength of this crystal will restore your vigour and your will to live. It promotes positive, pragmatic thought and sensible solutions, and can assist you to recognize the gifts that hide in the depths of your being.

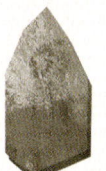

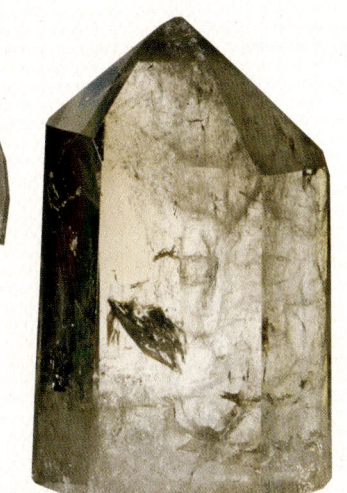

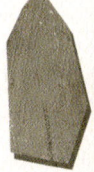

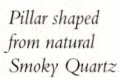

Pillar shaped from natural Smoky Quartz.

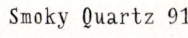

Emotions: Detoxifying and stabilizing your emotions, this is a stone of balance that teaches you how to leave behind anything that no longer serves you. It relieves fear, lifts depression, and induces emotional calmness. Smoky Quartz also aids acceptance of the physical body and resolves ambivalence.

Spirit: This crystal facilitates moving smoothly between alpha and beta states of mind (relaxation/daydreaming and wide-awake states) and assists in clearing the mind for meditation.

Curious fact: A large Smoky Quartz forms part of the Sceptre of Power of the Scottish royal regalia.

Did you know? This crystal was an essential ingredient of any magician's crystal toolkit. Dr Dee (1527–c.1608), Queen Elizabeth I's seer, owned a Smoky Quartz crystal "shewstone", which was used to guide the queen's decisions as to how to rule the country.

Hot tip: Place a large Smoky Quartz in your home to keep it energetically clean and well protected. Remember to cleanse the crystal regularly.

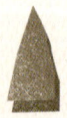
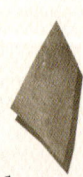
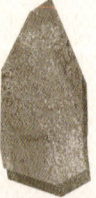

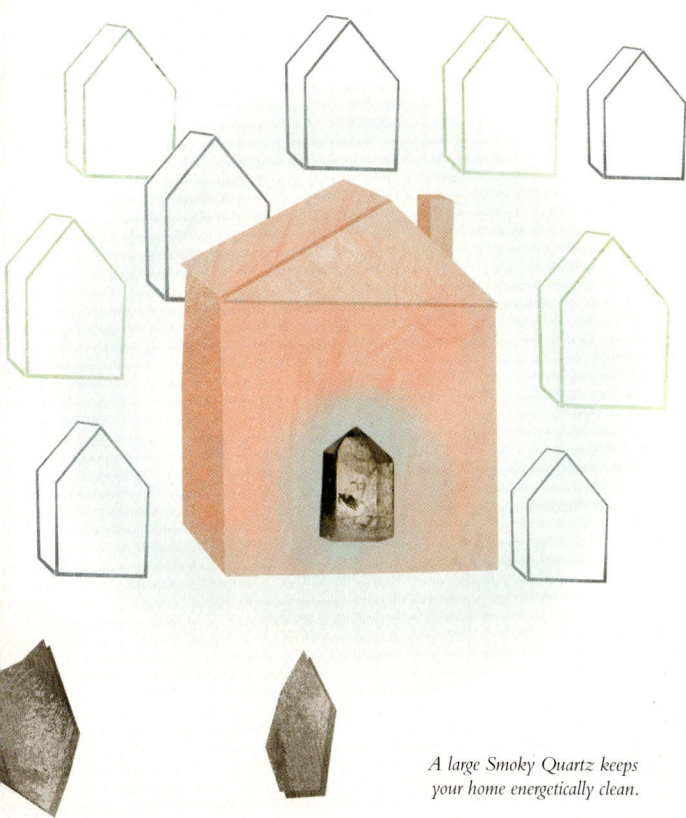

A large Smoky Quartz keeps your home energetically clean.

Smoky Quartz 93

Resources

Books by Judy Hall

101 Power Crystals: The ultimate guide to magical crystals, gems, and stones for healing and transformation (Quarto, UK; Fair Winds, USA)

Crystal Prescriptions: The A–Z guide to over 1,200 symptoms and their healing crystals, vols 1–4 (O-Books, UK and USA)

Crystals and Sacred Sites: Using crystals to harness the power of sacred landscapes (Quarto, UK; Fair Winds, USA)

Crystals for Psychic Self-Protection (Hay House, UK)

Crystals to Empower You (F&W Media Inc., USA)

Earth Blessing Crystals (Watkins Publishing, UK)

Good Vibrations: Energy enhancement, psychic protection and space clearing (Flying Horse Publications, UK)

Life-Changing Crystals: Using crystals to manifest abundance, wellbeing and happiness (Godsfield Press, UK)

The Crystal Bible, vols 1–3 (Godsfield Press, UK; Walking Stick Press, USA)

The Crystal Encyclopedia
(Godsfield Press, UK; Fair Winds, USA)

*The Crystal Experience: Your complete crystal workshop
in a book* (Godsfield Press, UK)

The Crystal Healing Pack (Godsfield Press, UK)

The Crystal Wisdom Oracle Pack (Watkins Publishing, UK)

"The Stone Horoscope: Evidence of continuity of ancient
esoteric tradition and practice. Are an authentic astrological
practice and archaic ideological narratives concatenating sky
and stones embedded in The Greek Alexander Romance?"
(MA dissertation, available at: www.judyhall.co.uk)

Crystals and Essences

Crystals attuned by Judy Hall are available from
www.angeladditions.co.uk

Exquisitecrystals.com is an online American retailer
that is highly recommended

Petaltone cleansing and recharging essences can
be obtained from www.petaltone.co.uk and
www.petaltoneusa.com

Picture credits

All photography copyright © Octopus Publishing Group.

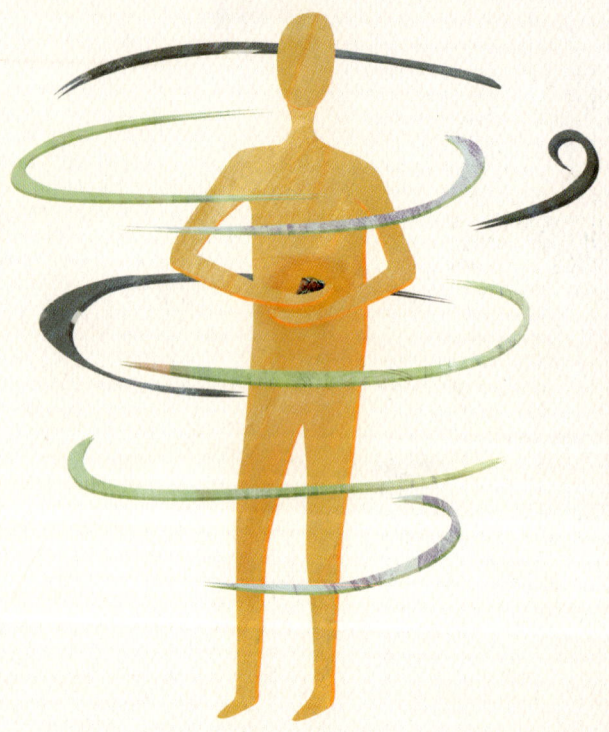